Falls in older people

Risk factors and strategies for prevention

Over the past two decades there has been a great deal of international, specialized research activity focused on risk factors and prevention strategies for falls in older people. This book provides health care workers with a detailed analysis of the most recent developments in the area and helps bridge the gap between scientific journal articles and general texts. The book is constructed in three parts: risk factors, prevention strategies, and future research directions. Coverage includes epidemiology, critical appraisal of the roles of exercise, environment, footwear, and medication, evidence-based risk assessment, and targeted and individually tailored falls-prevention strategies.

Falls in Older People will be invaluable to medical practitioners, physiotherapists, occupational therapists, nurses, researchers and all those working in community, hospital and residential aged care settings.

The authors are all based at Prince of Wales Medical Research Institute, Sydney.

Stephen R. Lord is a research fellow specializing in applied physiology, instability, risk factors and prevention of falls and fractures in older people. He also has conjoint academic appointments within the Schools of Community Medicine and Physiology and Pharmacology at the University of New South Wales and the Department of Aged Care, University of Sydney.

Catherine Sherrington is also a Senior Physiotherapist in Rehabilitation at Bankstown-Lidcombe Hospital in Sydney and cofounder of the Centre for Evidence-Based Physiotherapy at the University of Sydney.

Hylton B. Menz is also a lecturer in lower limb biomechanics and gerontology at the University of Western Sydney – Macarthur.

FALLS in older people

Risk factors and strategies for prevention

Stephen R. Lord
Prince of Wales Medical Research Institute, Sydney

Catherine Sherrington
Prince of Wales Medical Research Institute, Sydney

Hylton B. Menz
Prince of Wales Medical Research Institute, Sydney

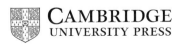

CAMBRIDGE
UNIVERSITY PRESS

PUBLISHED BY THE PRESS SYNDICATE OF THE UNIVERSITY OF CAMBRIDGE
The Pitt Building, Trumpington Street, Cambridge, United Kingdom

CAMBRIDGE UNIVERSITY PRESS
The Edinburgh Building, Cambridge CB2 2RU, UK
40 West 20th Street, New York, NY 10011–4211, USA
477 Williamstown Road, Port Melbourne, VIC 3207, Australia
Ruiz de Alarcón 13, 28014 Madrid, Spain
Dock House, The Waterfront, Cape Town 8001, South Africa

http://www.cambridge.org

First published 2001
Third printing 2004

Printed in the United Kingdom at the University Press, Cambridge

Typeface Minion 10.5/14pt   *System* QuarkXPress™   [s e]

A catalogue record for this book is available from the British Library

Library of Congress Cataloguing-in-Publication Data

Lord, Stephen R., 1957–
    Falls in older people : risk factors and strategies for prevention / by Stephen R. Lord,
    Catherine Sherrington, Hylton B. Menz.
        p. cm.
    Includes index.
    ISBN 0–521–58964–9 (pb)
    1. Falls (Accidents) in old age–Risk factors. 2. Falls (Accidents) in old
    age–Prevention. I. Sherrington, Catherine. II. Menz, Hylton B. III. Title.

    RC952.5 L67 2000
    617.1′0084′6–dc21   00–023656

ISBN 0 521 58964 9 paperback

Every effort has been made in preparing this book to provide accurate and up-to-date
information which is in accord with accepted standards and practice at the time of publication.
Nevertheless, the authors, editors and publisher can make no warranties that the information
contained herein is totally free from error, not least because clinical standards are constantly
changing through research and regulation. The authors, editors and publisher therefore
disclaim all liability for direct or consequential damages resulting from the use of material
contained in this book. Readers are strongly advised to pay careful attention to information
provided by the manufacturer of any drugs or equipment that they plan to use.

Contents

Part III   Research issues in falls prevention

Preface

In the last two decades of the twentieth century there was an enormous amount of work published in the international literature on risk factors for falling in older people and falls prevention strategies. The aim of this book is to review the material that has been published in specific journal articles to provide health care workers with a means for gaining access to contemporary findings. In doing so, we hope to bridge the gap between highly specialized journal articles and the often sketchy and superficial chapters on this topic that appear in many textbooks.

As suggested by the title, the book has two major themes: falls risk factors and falls prevention strategies. Part I includes an initial chapter on the epidemiology of falls and fall-related injuries in older people. Chapters 2 to 6 present critical appraisals of the many posited falls risk factors, addressed under the headings of postural stability, sensory and neuromuscular risk factors, medical risk factors, medications as risk factors, and environmental risk factors. In Chapter 7, the importance of the risk factors in each of the above domains is weighed as weak, moderate or strong, using evidence from published studies.

Part II addresses falls prevention strategies. An introductory overview outlines falls prevention strategies which address the multitude of falls risk factors. Chapters 8 to 11 examine the role of specific intervention strategies such as exercise, environmental modifications and the use of safe footwear, aids and appliances for preventing falls and falls injury. In Chapter 12, suggested strategies for preventing falls in institutions are summarized and discussed. Chapters 13 and 14 present clear guidelines for a systematic approach to the medical management of older persons at risk of falling, including management of medication use. The final two chapters of Part II focus on falls prevention strategies tailored to an individual's requirements. Chapter 15 summarizes the studies of targeted falls prevention strategies. Chapter 16 describes a novel profile system for quantifying an individual's risk of falling and targeting intervention strategies. Part III contains a single chapter which reviews the research issues that still need to be addressed in this field.

In each chapter we have attempted to be analytical in nature. Thus, we have not simply presented lists of the many and varied factors that have been suggested as possible but unproven risk factors for falls and the suggested but untested falls pre-vention strategies. Instead, we have attempted to evaluate the evidence for each factor implicated with falls to determine whether they constitute important areas for consideration and intervention. For example, we present arguments that chal-lenge some traditional approaches to the management of older persons at risk of falls. We question the utility of falls risk assessment based solely on diagnoses of disease processes and the value of standard clinical tests of vision, sensation, strength and balance. We also discuss the role of particular medications in predis-posing older people to falls and why factors such as alcohol use, vestibular disor-ders and postural hypotension (which are considered important risk factors in clinical practice) have not been demonstrated to be significant risk factors for falls in well-planned epidemiological studies. With regard to interventions, we examine the effectiveness of suggested strategies for preventing falls and question the value of interventions which do not take participant compliance issues into account.

As neurophysiological factors have been found to be key elements in the predic-tion and prevention of falls, this book places a major emphasis on these. Findings from our own studies have highlighted tests that have great utility in that they are reliable and highly predictive of falls. As outlined in Chapter 16, these tests can be used in a 'profile'-based approach to falls risk which is aimed at identifying specific impairments in the major sensorimotor systems that contribute to balance, i.e. vision, peripheral sensation, vestibular function, strength and reaction time as well as measures of sway and stability. This enables intervention strategies to be tailored to address an individual's specific deficits.

The length of the chapters in this book varies considerably. The longer chapters are in the areas in which there is a greater amount of available evidence on which to base falls risk factor assessment and the development of prevention strategies.

We hope this book will be of interest to medical and allied health care under-graduate and postgraduate students, medical practitioners, nurses, physiothera-pists, occupational therapists, podiatrists, research workers in the fields of gerontology and geriatrics, health service managers, scientists and health care workers in the disciplines of public health, injury and occupational health. We feel that this book is of relevance to those working in community, hospital, and resi-dential aged care settings.

Acknowledgements

The authors would like to acknowledge Beth Matters of the Prince of Wales Medical Research Institute, Sydney, for her entry on Chapter 5. We would also like to thank Dr Felicity Bagnall, Ms Joanne Corcoran, Dr Richard Fitzpatrick, Ms Lyn Gale, Dr Rob Herbert, Dr Sue Ogle, Ms Pat Pamphlett, Mr Karl Schurr, Ms Judy

Sherrington, Ms Amanda Wales and Dr John Ward for their thoughtful comments and contributions to various chapters of this book. Dr Jos Verbaken gave permission to reproduce the MET visual contrast chart. Professor John Campbell and Professor Bob Cumming forwarded prepublication versions of research articles, thus enabling the inclusion of important new material. Finally we would like to thank our partners and families for their support and tolerance throughout the writing process.

Part I

Risk factors for falls

Epidemiology of falls and fall-related injuries

In this chapter, we examine the epidemiology of falls in older people. We review the major studies that have described the incidence of falls, the locations where falls occur and falls sequelae. We also examine the costs and services required to treat and manage falls injuries. Before looking at the above, however, it is helpful to discuss briefly two important methodological considerations that are pertinent to all research studies of falls in older people. First, how falls are defined, and second, how falls are counted.

The definition of a fall

In 1987 the Kellogg International Working Group on the prevention of falls in the elderly defined a fall as 'unintentionally coming to the ground or some lower level and other than as a consequence of sustaining a violent blow, loss of consciousness, sudden onset of paralysis as in stroke or an epileptic seizure' [1]. Since then, many researchers have used this or very similar definitions of a fall. Depending on the focus of study, however, some researchers have used a broader definition of falls to include those that occur as a result of dizziness and syncope. The Kellogg definition is appropriate for studies aimed at identifying factors that impair sensorimotor function and balance control, whereas the broader definition is appropriate for studies that also address cardiovascular causes of falls such as postural hypotension and transient ischaemic attacks.

Although falls are often referred to as accidents, it has been shown statistically that falls incidence differs significantly from a Poisson distribution [2]. This implies that causal processes are involved in falls and that they are not merely random events.

Falls ascertainment

The earliest published studies on falls were retrospective in design in that they asked subjects whether and/or how many times they fell in a past period – usually 12 months. This approach has limitations because subjects have only limited accuracy in remembering falls over such a long period [3]. More recent studies have used prospective designs, in which subjects are followed up for a period, again usually 12 months, to determine more accurately the incidence of falling. Not surprisingly, these studies have usually reported higher rates of falling. In community studies, the only feasible method of ascertaining falls is by self-report and a number of methods have been used to record falls in prospective follow-up periods. These include monthly or bi-monthly mail-out questionnaires [4, 5], weekly [6] or monthly falls calendars [7], and monthly telephone interviews [8].

Each method has advantages and disadvantages in terms of accuracy, cost and researcher time commitment. Calendars have an advantage in that subjects are requested to indicate daily whether or not they have fallen. However, specific details about the circumstances of any falls cannot be ascertained until the diary is returned at the end of the month. Monthly questionnaires have an advantage in that all relevant details can be gained from a single form. A sample of a monthly questionnaire is shown in Figure 1.1. Telephone interviews gain the same information as mail-out questionnaires, but may require many calls to contact active older people. However, even with the most rigorous reporting methodology, it is quite likely that falls are underreported and that circumstances surrounding falls are sometimes incomplete or inaccurate. After a fall, older people are often shocked and distressed and may not remember the predisposing factors that led to the fall. Denial is also a factor in underreporting, as it is common for older people to lay the blame on external factors for their fall, and not count it as a 'true' one. Simply forgetting falls leads to further underreporting, especially in those with cognitive impairments.

In institutional settings, the use of falls record books maintained by nursing staff can provide an ancillary method for improving the accuracy of recording falls. In a study of intermediate care (hostel) residents in Sydney, we found that systematic recording of falls by nurses increased the number of falls reported by 32% [4].

The incidence of falls in older people

Community-dwellers

In 1977, Exton-Smith examined the incidence of falls in 963 people over the age of 65 years. He found that in women, the proportion who fell increased with age from about 30% in the 65–69 year age group to over 50% in those over the age of 85 years. In men, the proportion who fell increased from 13% in the 65–69 year age group to levels of approximately 30% in those aged 80 years and over [9].

Retrospective community studies undertaken since Exton-Smith's work have reported similar findings: that about 30% of older persons experience one or more

---

FALLS STUDY OCTOBER FOLLOW-UP

1. HAVE YOU HAD ANY FALLS IN THE MONTH OF OCTOBER?

I have not fallen	[ ]
Once	[ ]
Twice	[ ]
Three or more times	[ ]

If you have had <u>no falls</u> please stop here, otherwise please continue

2. WHERE HAVE YOU FALLEN?

<u>Inside</u>:

On the one level	Yes [ ]	No	[ ]
Getting out of bed	Yes [ ]	No	[ ]
Getting out of a chair	Yes [ ]	No	[ ]
Using the shower/bath	Yes [ ]	No	[ ]
Using the toilet	Yes [ ]	No	[ ]
Walking up or down stairs	Yes [ ]	No	[ ]

<u>Home entrances or in the garden</u>:

Walking up or down a step/stairs			
On the one level (e.g. pathway)	Yes [ ]	No	[ ]
In the garden	Yes [ ]	No	[ ]

<u>Away from home</u>:

On the footpath	Yes [ ]	No	[ ]
On a kerb / gutter	Yes [ ]	No	[ ]
In a public building	Yes [ ]	No	[ ]
Getting out of a vehicle	Yes [ ]	No	[ ]
In another person's home	Yes [ ]	No	[ ]

Falls not described above (Please specify)

_____

3. HOW DID YOU FALL?
(Tick more than one if necessary)

I tripped	[ ]
I slipped	[ ]
I lost my balance	[ ]
My legs gave way	[ ]
I felt faint	[ ]
I felt giddy / dizzy	[ ]
I am not sure	[ ]

4. AS A RESULT OF THIS FALL OR FALLS DID YOU SUFFER ANY INJURIES?

Yes [ ]   No [ ]

5. IF YES WHAT TYPE OF INJURIES DID YOU SUFFER?

Bruises	[ ]
Cuts/grazes	[ ]
Broken wrist	[ ]
Broken hip	[ ]
Broken ribs	[ ]
Back pain	[ ]

Thank you very much for your co-operation. Please return the questionnaire to us by using the enclosed envelope

Fig. 1.1.   Example of a monthly falls questionnaire.

falls per year [10–12]. For example, Campbell et al. [10] analysed a stratified population sample of 533 subjects aged 65 years and over and found that 33% experienced one or more falls in the past year. Blake et al. [12] reported a similar incidence (35%) in their study of 1042 subjects aged 65 years and over. In a large study of 2793 subjects aged 65 years and over, Prudham and Evans [11] estimated an annual incidence for accidental falls of 28%, a figure identical to that found in the Dubbo osteoporosis epidemiology study of 1762 older people aged 60 years and over [13].

More recent prospective studies undertaken in community settings have found slightly higher falls incidence rates. In the Randwick falls and fractures study conducted in Australia, we found that 39% of 341 community-dwelling women reported one or more falls in a 1-year follow-up period [14]. In a large study of 761 subjects aged 70 years and over undertaken in New Zealand, Campbell et al. [15] found that 40% of 465 women and 28% of 296 men fell at least once in the study period of 1 year, an overall incidence rate of 35%.

In the USA, Tinetti et al. [7] found an incidence rate of one or more falls of 32% in 336 subjects aged 75 years and over. Similar rates have been reported in Canada by O'Loughlin et al. [8] in a 48-week prospective study of a random sample of 409 community-dwelling people aged 65 + years (29%), and in Finland by Luukinen et al. [16] in 833 community-dwelling people aged 70 + years from five rural districts (30%). Falling rates also increase beyond the age of 65 years. Figure 1.2 shows the proportion of women who took part in the Randwick falls and fractures study [14] who reported falling, once, twice, or three or more times in a 12-month period.

The prospective studies that have reported the incidence of multiple or recurrent falls are also in good agreement. The reported rates from five studies for two or more falls in follow-up year average 15% and range from 11% to 21%. The three studies that report data for three or more falls all report an incidence of 8%.

Residents of long-term care institutions

Studies on the prevalence of falls have also been conducted in institutions, where the reported frequency of falling is considerably higher than among those living in their own homes. For example, Luukinen et al. [17] estimate that among people aged 70 and over in Finland, the rate of falling in the institutionalized population is three times higher than that among those living independently in the community.

The prospective studies conducted in nursing homes have found 12-month falls incidence rates ranging from 30% to 56%. In an early study, Fernie et al. [18] studied 205 nursing home residents for 12 months and found 30% of the men and 42% of the women had one or more falls. More recently, two studies have reported higher falls incidence rates in institutionalized older people. Lipsitz et al. [19] found

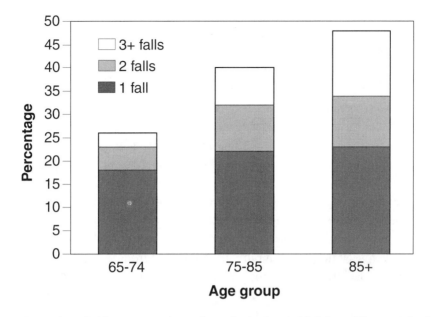

Fig. 1.2.   Proportion of older women who took part in the Randwick Falls and Fractures Study who reported falling, once, twice or three or more times in a 12-month period. Diagram adapted from: Lord SR, Ward JA, Williams P, Anstey KJ. An epidemiological study of falls in older community-dwelling women: the Randwick falls and fractures study. *Australian Journal of Public Health* 1993;17(3):240–5.

that 40% of 901 ambulatory nursing home residents fell two or more times in 6 months and Yip and Cumming [20] found that 56% of 126 nursing home residents fell at least once in a year.

Two other studies have calculated falls incidence rates across a number of nursing homes. Rubenstein et al. [21] summarized the findings from five published and two unpublished studies on the incidence of falls in long-term care institutions. They calculated that the incidence rate ranged between 60% to 290% per bed, with a mean fall incidence rate of 170% or 1.7 falls per person per year. Thapa et al. [22] conducted a 12-month prospective study in 12 nursing homes involving 1228 residents. They reported that during the 1003 person-years of follow-up, 548 residents suffered 1585 falls.

Falling rates are also high in residents living in intermediate (hostel) care institutions and retirement villages. We found a yearly falls incidence rate for one or more falls of 52%, and for two or more falls of 39% in a hostel population of older people [4]. Tinetti et al. [23] also found a high incidence of falling in 79 persons admitted consecutively to intermediate care facilities: 32% fell two or more times in a 3-month period. In the one study that has been conducted in a retirement village to date, Liu et al. [24] found that 61% of 96 subjects fell over a 12-month period.

Particular groups

Older people who have suffered a fall are at increased risk of falling again. In a prospective study of 325 community-dwelling persons who had fallen in the previous year, Nevitt et al. [6] found that 57% experienced at least one fall in a 12-month follow-up period and 31% had two or more falls. Not surprisingly, falling is also more prevalent in frailer older people than vigorous ones, in those who have difficulties undertaking activities of daily living, and in those with particular medical conditions that affect posture, balance and gait. Northridge et al. [25] reported that when community-dwelling persons were classified as either frail or vigorous, frailer people were more than twice as likely to fall as vigorous people. Similarly, Speechley and Tinetti [26] reported 52% of a frail group fell in a 1-year prospective period compared with only 17% of a vigorous group.

With regard to medical conditions, Mahoney et al. [27] found that 14% of older patients fell in the first month after discharge from hospital following a medical illness. Falling rates are also increased in those with stroke and Parkinson's disease. Forster and Young [28] found that 73% of elderly stroke patients fell within 6 months after hospital discharge. Koller et al. [29] and Paulson et al. [30] report falling yearly incidence rates of 38% and 53% respectively in elderly people with idiopathic Parkinson's disease. Kroller et al. [29] also noted that very frequent falling was a problem in this group, with 13% reporting falling more than once a week. Falls incidence is also high in older people following lower limb amputation. Kulkarni [31] found that 58% of people with a unilateral amputation had at least one fall within a 12-month period before their survey.

Increased falls incidence is also evident in persons with cognitive impairments and other neurological conditions, arthritis and diabetes, although few studies have reported specific falls incidence rates in these groups. In one study that examined falls incidence in persons with Alzheimer's disease, only 17% were reported to fall within a prospective period of 3 years [32]. This would appear to be an underestimate, as cognitive impairment has been found to be an independent risk factor for falling in many subsequent prospective studies (see Chapter 4).

Falls location

In independent older community-dwelling people, about 50% of falls occur within their homes and immediate home surroundings (Figure 1.3) [16, 33]. Most falls occur on level surfaces within commonly used rooms such as the bedroom, living-room and kitchen. Comparatively few falls occur in the bathroom, on stairs or from ladders and stools. While a proportion of falls involve a hazard such as a loose rug or a slippery floor, many do not involve obvious environmental hazards [33]. The remaining falls occur in public places and other people's homes. Commonly

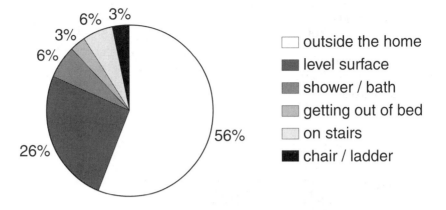

Fig. 1.3.   Location of falls. 56% of falls occur outside the home (in the garden, street, footpath or shops), with the remainder (44%) occurring at various locations in the home. Adapted from: Lord SR, Ward JA, Williams P, Anstey KJ. Physiological factors associated with falls in older community-dwelling women. *Australian Journal of Public Health* 1993;17(3):240–5.

reported environmental factors involved in falls in public places include pavement cracks and misalignments, gutters, steps, construction works, uneven ground and slippery surfaces.

The location of falls is related to age, sex and frailty. In community-dwelling older women, we found that the number of falls occurring outside the home decreased with age, with a corresponding increase in the number of falls occurring inside the home on a level surface (Figure 1.4) [14]. Campbell et al. [33] found that fewer men than women fell inside the home (44% versus 65%) and more men fell in the garden (25% versus 11%). Also as would be expected, frailer groups with limited mobility suffer most falls within the home. These findings indicate that the occurrence of falls is strongly related to exposure, that is, they occur in situations where older people are undertaking their usual daily activities. Furthermore, most falls occur during periods of maximum activity in the morning or afternoon, and only about 20% occur between 9 p.m. and 7 a.m. [33].

Consequences of falls

Falls are the leading cause of injury-related hospitalization in persons aged 65 years and over, and account for 4% of all hospital admissions in this age group [34]. In Australia we found that hospital admissions resulting from falls are uncommon in young adulthood but with advancing age, the incidence of fall-related admissions increases at an exponential rate. Beyond 40 years, the admission rate due to falls increases consistently by 4.5% per year for men (doubling every 15.7 years) and by 7.9% per year for women (doubling every 9.1 years) [35] (Figure 1.5). In those aged

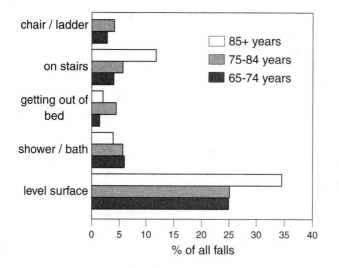

Fig. 1.4.   Indoor falls location according to age. Adapted from: Lord SR, Ward JA, Williams P, Anstey KJ. An epidemiological study of falls in older community-dwelling women: the Randwick falls and fractures study. *Australian Journal of Public Health* 1993;17(3):240–5.

85 years and over, the levels have reached 4% per annum in men and 7% per annum in women. Falls also account for 40% of injury-related deaths, and 1% of total deaths in this age group [36].

Depending on the population under study, between 22% and 60% of older people suffer injuries from falls, 10–15% suffer serious injuries, 2–6% suffer fractures and 0.2–1.5% suffer hip fractures. The most commonly self-reported injuries include superficial cuts and abrasions, bruises and sprains. The most common injuries that require hospitalization comprise femoral neck fractures, other fractures of the leg, fractures of radius, ulna and other bones in the arm and fractures of the neck and trunk [1, 26, 35].

In terms of morbidity and mortality, the most serious of these fall-related injuries is fracture of the hip. Elderly people recover slowly from hip fractures and are vulnerable to postoperative complications. In many cases, hip fractures result in death and of those who survive, many never regain complete mobility. Marottoli et al. [37] analysed the outcomes of 120 patients from a cohort study who suffered a hip fracture over a 6-year period. They found that before their fractures, 86% could dress independently, 75% could walk independently and 63% could climb a flight of stairs. Six months after their injuries, these percentages had fallen to 49%, 15% and 8%, respectively.

Another consequence of falling is the 'long lie', i.e. remaining on the ground or floor for more than an hour after a fall. The long lie is a marker of weakness, illness and social isolation and is associated with high mortality rates among the

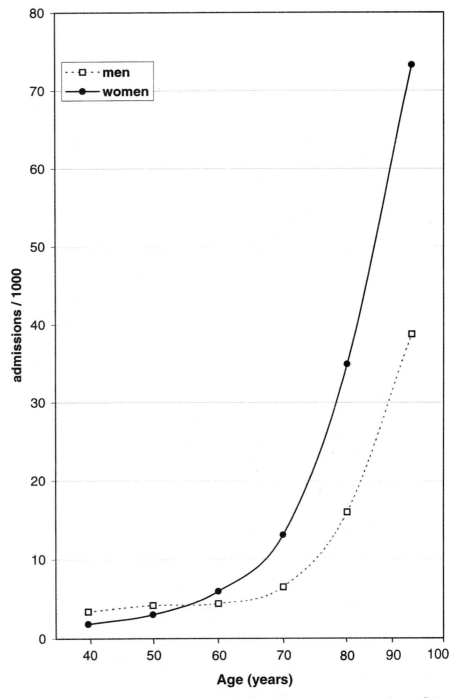

Fig. 1.5.   Hospital admissions for falls according to age and gender. Adapted from: Lord SR. Falls in the elderly: admissions, bed use, outcome and projections. *Medical Journal of Australia* 1990;153:117–18.

elderly. Time spent on the floor is associated with fear of falling, muscle damage, pneumonia, pressure sores, dehydration and hypothermia [6, 38, 39]. Wild et al. [40] found that half of those who lie on the floor for an hour or longer die within 6 months, even if there is no direct injury from the fall. Vellas [41] suggests that long lies are not uncommon. He found that more than 20% of patients admitted to hospital because of a fall had been on the ground for an hour or more. Such a figure could be expected as Tinetti et al. [42] found that up to 47% of non-injured fallers are unable to get up off the floor without assistance.

Falls can result in restriction of activity and fear of falling, reduced quality of life and independence. Even falls that do not result in physical injuries can result in the 'post-fall syndrome'; a loss of confidence, hesitancy, tentativeness, with resultant loss of mobility and independence. It has been found that after falling, 48% of older people report a fear of falling and 25% report curtailing activities [6, 43]. Tinetti et al. [43] have also found that 15% of nonfallers also report avoiding activities due to a fear of falling.

Finally, falls can also lead to disability and decreased mobility which often results in increased dependency on others and hence an increased probability of being admitted to an institution. Falls are commonly cited as a contributing reason for an older person requiring admission to a nursing home [42, 44].

The cost of falls

As indicated above, falls in older people are common and can lead to numerous disabling conditions, extensive hospital stays and death. It is not at all surprising, then, that falls constitute a significant health care cost. Fall-related costs can include the direct costs, which include doctor visits, acute hospital and nursing home care, outpatient clinics, rehabilitation stays, diagnostic tests, medications, home care, home modifications, equipment and institutional care. Indirect costs include carer and patient morbidity and mortality costs. The literature on the total cost of falls is scarce, however, as there are many difficulties and limitations involved in estimating the economic cost of any disease or condition. Problems exist because cost data are only estimates, and many costs are only relevant to the country in which they are incurred. Furthermore, because of inflation and other economic and health care factors, costs are outdated soon after they are published.

A number of researchers have estimated the hospital costs of an injurious fall in absolute terms and as a proportion of health budgets [35, 45–49]. In a detailed report to the US Congress in 1989, Rice and MacKenzie [48] calculated that in 1985, nearly $10 billion of the $158 billion or 6% of the lifetime economic cost of injury in the United States was attributable to falls in older people. Furthermore, falls account for 70% of all injury-related costs in elderly people. The cost per injured person in 1985 was $4226, which was nearly double that of the average cost per injured person for all age groups. Englander et al. [49] updated the costs of falls as presented by Rice and MacKenzie [48] from 1985 US dollars to 1994 US dollars. They projected the cost of falls in 1994 to total $20.2 billion, with a cost per injured person being $7399. The authors further extrapolated these figures to the year 2020 and estimated the cost of falls injuries at $32.4 billion.

Conclusion

Despite the disparate methodologies of falls ascertainment used in the above studies, the incidence rates reported are remarkably similar. Approximately one third of older people living in the community fall at least once a year, with many suffering multiple falls. Falling rates are higher in older women (40%) than in older men (28%) and continue to increase with age above 65 years. The incidence of falls is increased in people living in retirement villages, hostels and nursing homes, in those who have fallen in the past year and in those with particular medical conditions that affect posture, balance and gait. In community-dwelling older people, about 50% of falls occur within their homes and 50% in public places. Falls account for 4% of hospital admissions, 40% of injury-related deaths and 1% of total deaths in persons aged 65 years and over. The major injuries that result from falls include fractures of the wrist, neck, trunk and hip. Falls can also result in disability, restriction of activity and fear of falling, which can reduce quality of life and independence and contribute to an older person being admitted to a nursing home. Finally, as many fall-related injuries require medical treatment including hospitalization, falls constitute a condition requiring considerable health care expenditure.

REFERENCES

1 Gibson MJ, Andres RO, Isaacs B, Radebaugh T, Worm-Petersen J. The prevention of falls in later life. A report of the Kellogg International Work Group on the prevention of falls by the elderly. *Danish Medical Bulletin* 1987;34(Suppl 4):1–24.

2 Grimley-Evans J. Fallers, non-fallers and Poisson. *Age and Ageing* 1990;19:268–9.

3 Cummings SR, Nevitt MC, Kidd S. Forgetting falls. The limited accuracy of recall of falls in the elderly. *Journal of the American Geriatrics Society* 1988;36:613–16.

4 Lord SR, Clark RD, Webster IW. Physiological factors associated with falls in an elderly population. *Journal of the American Geriatrics Society* 1991;39:1194–200.

5 Lord SR, Ward JA, Williams P, Anstey KJ. Physiological factors associated with falls in older community-dwelling women. *Journal of the American Geriatrics Society* 1994;42:1110–17.

6 Nevitt MC, Cummings SR, Kidd S, Black D: Risk factors for recurrent nonsyncopal falls. A prospective study. *Journal of the American Medical Association* 1989;261:2663–8.

7 Tinetti ME, Speechley M, Ginter SF. Risk factors for falls among elderly persons living in the community. *New England Journal of Medicine* 1988;319:1701–7.

8 O'Loughlin JL, Robitaille Y, Boivin JF, Suissa S. Incidence of and risk factors for falls and injurious falls among the community-dwelling elderly. *American Journal of Epidemiology* 1993;137:342–54.

9 Exton-Smith AN. Functional consequences of ageing: clinical manifestations. In Exton-Smith AN, Grimley Evans J editors. *Care of the elderly: meeting the challenge of dependency.* London: Academic Press, 1977.

10 Campbell AJ, Reinken J, Allan BC, Martinez GS. Falls in old age: a study of frequency and related clinical factors. *Age and Ageing* 1981;10:264–70.

11 Prudham D, Evans JG. Factors associated with falls in the elderly: a community study. *Age and Ageing* 1981;10:141–6.

12 Blake A, Morgan K, Bendall M, et al. Falls by elderly people at home: prevalence and associated factors. *Age and Ageing* 1988;17:365–72.

13 Lord SR, Sambrook PN, Gilbert C, et al. Postural stability, falls and fractures in the elderly: results from the Dubbo osteoporosis epidemiology study. *Medical Journal of Australia* 1994;160:684–5, 688–91.

14 Lord SR, Ward JA, Williams P, Anstey KJ. An epidemiological study of falls in older community-dwelling women: the Randwick falls and fractures study. *Australian Journal of Public Health* 1993;17:240–5.

15 Campbell AJ, Borrie MJ, Spears GF. Risk factors for falls in a community-based prospective study of people 70 years and older. *Journal of Gerontology* 1989;44:M112–17.

16 Luukinen H, Koski K, Laippala P, Kivela SL. Predictors for recurrent falls among the home-dwelling elderly. *Scandinavian Journal of Primary Health Care* 1995;13:294–9.

17 Luukinen H, Koski K, Hiltunen L, Kivela SL. Incidence rate of falls in an aged population in northern Finland. *Journal of Clinical Epidemiology* 1994;47:843–50.

18 Fernie GR, Gryfe CI, Holliday PJ, Llewellyn A. The relationship of postural sway in standing to the incidence of falls in geriatric subjects. *Age and Ageing* 1982;11:11–16.

19 Lipsitz LA, Jonsson PV, Kelley MM, Koestner JS. Causes and correlates of recurrent falls in ambulatory frail elderly. *Journal of Gerontology* 1991;46:M114–22.

20 Yip YB, Cumming RG: The association between medications and falls in Australian nursing-home residents. *Medical Journal of Australia* 1994;160:14–18.

21 Rubenstein LZ, Robbins AS, Schulman BL, Rosado J, Osterweil D, Josephson KR. Falls and instability in the elderly [clinical conference]. *Journal of the American Geriatrics Society* 1988;36:266–78.

22 Thapa PB, Brockman KG, Gideon P, Fought RL, Ray WA. Injurious falls in nonambulatory nursing home residents: a comparative study of circumstances, incidence, and risk factors. *Journal of the American Geriatrics Society* 1996;44:273–8.

23 Tinetti ME, Williams TF, Mayewski R. Fall risk index for elderly patients based on number of chronic disabilities. *American Journal of Medicine* 1986;80:429–34.

24 Liu BA, Topper AK, Reeves RA, Gryfe C, Maki BE. Falls among older people: relationship to medication use and orthostatic hypotension. *Journal of the American Geriatrics Society* 1995;43:1141–5.

25 Northridge ME, Nevitt MC, Kelsey JL, Link B. Home hazards and falls in the elderly: the role of health and functional status. *American Journal of Public Health* 1995;85:509–15.

26 Speechley M, Tinetti M. Falls and injuries in frail and vigorous community elderly persons. *Journal of the American Geriatrics Society* 1991;39:46–52.

27 Mahoney J, Sager M, Dunham NC, Johnson J. Risk of falls after hospital discharge. *Journal of the American Geriatrics Society* 1994;42:269–74.

28 Forster A, Young J. Incidence and consequences of falls due to stroke: a systematic inquiry. *British Medical Journal* 1995; 311:83–6.

29 Koller WC, Glatt S, Vetere-Overfield B, Hassanein R. Falls and Parkinson's disease. *Clinical Neuropharmacology* 1989;12:98–105.

30 Paulson GW, Schaefer K, Hallum B. Avoiding mental changes and falls in older Parkinson's patients. *Geriatrics* 1986;41:59–62.

31 Kulkarni J, Toole C, Hirons R, Wright S, Morris J. Falls in patients with lower limb amputations: prevalence and contributing factors. *Physiotherapy* 1996;82:130–6.

32 Buchner DM, Larson EB. Falls and fractures in patients with Alzheimer-type dementia. *Journal of the American Medical Association* 1987;257:1492–5.

33 Campbell AJ, Borrie MJ, Spears GF, Jackson SL, Brown JS, Fitzgerald JL. Circumstances and consequences of falls experienced by a community population 70 years and over during a prospective study. *Age and Ageing* 1990;19:136–41.

34 Baker SP, Harvey AH. Fall injuries in the elderly. *Clinics in Geriatric Medicine* 1985; 1:501–12.

35 Lord SR. Falls in the elderly: admissions, bed use, outcome and projections. *Medical Journal of Australia* 1990;153:117–18.

36 New South Wales Health Department: The epidemiology of falls in older people in NSW. Sydney: New South Wales Health Department, 1994.

37 Marottoli RA, Berkman LF, Cooney LM Jr. Decline in physical function following hip fracture. *Journal of the American Geriatrics Society* 1992;40:861–6.

38 Mallinson W, Green M. Covert muscle injury in aged persons admitted to hospital following falls. *Age and Ageing* 1985;14:174–8.

39 King MB, Tinetti ME. Falls in community-dwelling older persons. *Journal of the American Geriatrics Society* 1995;43:1146–54.

40 Wild D, Nayak US, Isaacs B. How dangerous are falls in old people at home? *British Medical Journal (Clinical Research)* 1981;282:266–8.

41 Vellas B, Cayla F, Bocquet H, de Pemille F, Albarede JL. Prospective study of restriction of activity in old people after falls. *Age and Ageing* 1987;16:189–93.

42 Tinetti ME, Liu WL, Claus EB. Predictors and prognosis of inability to get up after falls among elderly persons. *Journal of the American Medical Association* 1993;269:65–70.

43 Tinetti ME, Mendes de Leon CF, Doucette JT, Baker DI. Fear of falling and fall-related efficacy in relationship to functioning among community-living elders. *Journal of Gerontology* 1994;49:M140–7.

44 Lord SR. Predictors of nursing home placement and mortality of residents in intermediate care. *Age and Ageing* 1994;23:499–504.

45 Alexander BH, Rivara FP, Wolf ME. The cost and frequency of hospitalization for fall-related injuries in older adults. *American Journal of Public Health* 1992;82:1020–3.

46 Covington DL, Maxwell JG, Clancy TV. Hospital resources used to treat the injured elderly at North Carolina trauma centers. *Journal of the American Geriatrics Society* 1993;41:847–52.

47 Sjogren H, Bjornstig U. Unintentional injuries among elderly people: incidence, causes, severity, and costs. *Accident Analysis and Prevention* 1989;21:233–42.

48 Rice DP, MacKenzie EJ. *Cost of injury in the United States: a report to Congress.* San Francisco: Institute for Health and Ageing, University of California, 1989.

49 Englander F, Hodson TJ, Terregrossa RA. Economic dimensions of slip and fall injuries. *Journal of Forensic Sciences* 1996;41:733–46.

2

Postural stability and falls

Postural stability can be defined as the ability of an individual to maintain the position of the body, or more specifically, its centre of mass, within specific boundaries of space, referred to as *stability limits*. Stability limits are boundaries in which the body can maintain its position without changing the base of support [1]. This definition of postural stability is useful as it highlights the need to discuss stability in the context of a particular task or activity. For example, the stability limit of normal relaxed standing is the area bounded by the two feet on the ground, whereas the stability limit of unipedal stance is reduced to the area covered by the single foot in contact with the ground. Due to this reduction in the size of the stability limit, unipedal stance is an inherently more challenging task requiring greater postural control.

Regardless of the task being performed, maintaining postural stability requires the complex integration of sensory information regarding the position of the body relative to the surroundings, and the ability to generate forces to control body movement. Thus, postural stability requires the interaction of musculoskeletal and sensory systems. The musculoskeletal component of postural stability encompasses the biomechanical properties of body segments, muscles and joints. The sensory components include vision, vestibular function and somatosensation which act to inform the brain of the position and movement of the body in three-dimensional space. Linking these two components together are the higher-level neurological processes enabling anticipatory mechanisms responsible for planning a movement, and adaptive mechanisms responsible for the ability to react to changing demands of the particular task [1].

Normal ageing is associated with changes in function of each of the sub-components of musculoskeletal and sensory systems which contribute to postural stability [2–5]. Consequently ageing may manifest as a measurable deficit in any task involving maintaining postural stability. This chapter reviews the available literature regarding age-associated changes in postural stability for a number of specific tasks.

Postural stability when standing

Normal relaxed standing is characterized by small amounts of *postural sway* (also referred to as *body sway*), which has been defined by Sheldon as 'the constant small deviations from the vertical and their subsequent correction to which all human beings are subject when standing upright' [6]. Control of postural sway when standing involves continual muscle activity (primarily of the calf muscles) and requires an integrated reflex response to visual, vestibular and somatosensory inputs [7]. The significance of each of these systems has been determined by experimentally blocking each of these inputs and assessing subsequent postural sway. The role of vision has been assessed by simply asking the subjects to close their eyes, vestibular input has been minimized by tilting the head [8] or assessing the ability of subjects to balance an equivalent mechanical body [9], and somatosensory input has been blocked by ischaemia [7], standing on compliant surfaces [10, 11] and immersing the feet in cold water [12–14]. Numerous investigations have revealed that if any of these inputs are removed, postural sway increases. Although the extent to which one input can compensate for the loss of another is unclear, there is some evidence that peripheral sensation is the most important sensory system in the regulation of standing balance in older adults [11].

The generalized decline in sensory functions due to normal ageing and its contribution to increased postural sway have been widely evaluated in the literature. Although interest in the measurement of sway dates back to the classic studies on tabes dorsalis by Romberg in 1853 [15], the first attempt to assess age-related changes in postural sway was conducted by Hellebrandt and Braun in 1939 [16], who measured subjects aged from 3 to 86 years. The results showed that the magnitude of sway was largest in the very young and very old subjects. A similar study by Boman and Jalavisto [17] measured sway with an overhead camera in subjects aged 18–30 and 61–88 years, and reported that sway was greater in the elderly group, particularly in those aged over 80 years.

Since these early investigations, a large number of studies have reported age-associated increases in standing postural sway after the age of 30 years using various sway meters, optical systems and force platforms, particularly when subjects close their eyes [5, 6, 18–40]. There is no clear consensus in the literature regarding gender differences in sway; although some studies report higher postural sway values in women compared with men in all age groups [18, 21, 24], other authors have reported no significant differences [27, 29, 35, 41].

Factors found to be highly correlated with increased sway include reduced lower extremity muscle strength [11, 42–44], reduced peripheral sensation [22, 23, 45–48], poor near visual acuity [11, 49] and slowed reaction time [11, 50]. We have previously found that while reaction time is not associated with sway when standing on a firm surface, when subjects stand on a compliant foam rubber surface a significant association between sway and reaction time is evident [11]. This suggests that subjects can perceive large amounts of sway and therefore consciously react to control their body movements. Smaller associations between vestibular function and sway have been reported [8, 11, 22, 51]. The role of these physiological systems in contributing to falls is further discussed in Chapter 3.

Body morphology and alignment have not been widely evaluated. Danis et al. [52] reported that skeletal alignment was not closely associated with postural sway on a force plate, however Lichtenstein et al. [49] and Era et al. [43] reported that low body mass is associated with greater sway in both men and women.

Measurement of postural sway when standing has been reported to be a useful predictor of falls in older people. These investigations have taken two forms: cross-sectional studies, which classify subjects as 'fallers' or 'nonfallers' based on self-reported previous history of experiencing a fall, and prospective studies, which measure balance variables among a group of subjects and then follow them over a period of time to delineate fallers from nonfallers. A number of cross-sectional studies have reported significantly greater sway in subjects with a history of falling compared to nonfallers [21, 41, 53, 54]. Similarly, prospective studies have revealed that the measurement of an individual's sway is a useful predictor of the risk of falling during follow-up periods [55–59].

In our studies we have found that fallers show greater sway in four test conditions: standing on a firm base with the eyes open; standing on a firm base with the eyes closed; standing on 15-cm-thick medium-density foam rubber with the eyes open; and standing on the foam rubber with the eyes closed [55, 60–62]. In each of these studies, we have used a specially designed, portable sway-meter which records the displacements of the body at the level of the waist (see Figure 2.1). We have also noted that an inability to maintain balance on the foam at all is associated with falling.

In addition to the investigation of standing postural sway, a number of other standing tests have been developed which provide a greater challenge to the postural control system. One technique for further challenging the postural control system is simply to alter foot position, thereby decreasing the size of the stability limit. This concept was first explored by Romberg [15], who assessed balance by observing the ability of patients to stand with their feet together. The effect of foot position on sway has more recently been evaluated in detail by numerous authors [63–66], who evaluated postural stability on a force plate with subjects standing with their feet in varying positions (i.e.: toe-in, toe-out, variations in space between the heels and tandem stance). Increased sway was apparent with the more challenging conditions due to the reduction in the size of the stability limit. In accordance with investigations into normal bipedal standing, ageing is also associated

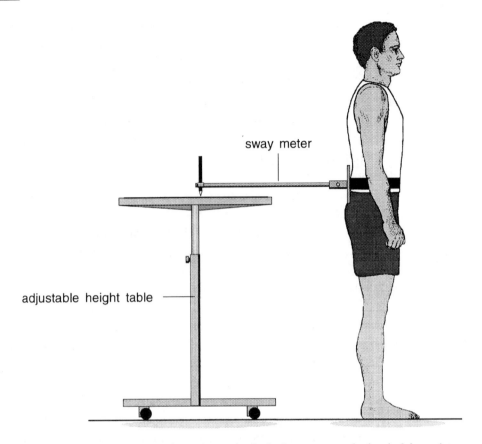

sway meter

adjustable height table

Fig. 2.1.   The portable 'sway meter' used to measure body displacements at the level of the waist.

with poorer performance in tandem standing [44, 67–71] and unipedal stance [18, 23, 24, 68–70, 72–76]. In a recently completed study, we found that older people with a history of falls had increased lateral sway with the eyes open and closed when undertaking a near-tandem stability test. The fallers were also significantly more likely to take a protective step when undertaking the test with the eyes closed [77]. Similarly, three studies have reported that performance in the unipedal standing test is also capable of predicting falls in older people [72, 76, 78].

Postural stability during leaning tasks

An alternative approach to challenge postural control is to measure sway when the subject is placed at the perimeter of their stability limit, or to measure the dimensions of the stability limit itself. Hasselkus and Shambes [20] assessed postural sway in young and older women in normal relaxed stance and when the subjects leaned forward at the waist approximately 45 degrees. The results revealed that sway was greater in the older group in both conditions, but particularly so when leaning forward, suggesting that the older women were less able to stabilize their posture when approaching the perimeter of their stability limit. King et al. [79] evaluated the ability of women aged 20–91 years to reach as far forward and backward as possible when standing, in order to establish age-related differences in functional base of support. Decreased functional base of support was evident after the age of 60 years, and declined 16% per decade thereafter.

A similar technique is the *functional reach test*, which involves the measurement of a subject's ability to reach forward as far as possible with the arm positioned at 90 degrees of shoulder flexion. This test was first described by Duncan et al. [80], who evaluated subjects aged 21–87 years and reported a significant age-related decline in functional reach. Similar results were reported by Hagemon [35], who reported that older subjects exhibited a smaller mean reach than younger subjects. Subsequent investigations of functional reach have shown the test to be correlated with performance in activities of daily living [81], a predictor of falls [82], and sensitive to improvements in function following rehabilitation [83]. However, a recent investigation by Wernick-Robin et al. [84] suggested that functional reach is not a valid indicator of dynamic balance, due to the variety of strategies that can be used to extend the arm from the shoulder. A different technique was employed by Thelen et al. [85] in which young and older subjects were held in a harness in a forward-leaning position and their responses to the release of the harness support observed. Older subjects could only regain balance from relatively small initial leaning positions compared with the younger subjects, further suggesting that the ability to control the centre of mass diminishes with age.

We have developed two additional standing tests as measures of postural stability [86]. The *maximum balance range* test involves the subject leaning forward and backward from the ankles as far as possible (without moving their feet or bending at the hips). Maximal anteroposterior distance moved is measured using a pen attached to a rod extending anteriorly from the subject's waist. This technique provides some benefits over the functional reach test, as it avoids problems associated with variations in shoulder movement when extending the arm. The pen records the anterior and posterior movements of the subject on a sheet of graph paper which is fastened to the top of an adjustable height table. Using a similar apparatus, an additional test of *coordinated stability* can be performed in which the subject is asked to adjust body position by bending or rotating the body without moving the feet so that the pen on the end of the rod follows and remains within a convoluted track marked on a piece of paper attached to the top of an adjustable height table. To complete the test without errors, subjects have to remain within the track, which is 1.5 cm wide, and be capable of adjusting the position of the pen 29 cm laterally and 18 cm in the anteroposterior plane. A total error score is calculated by summing the number of occasions that the pen on the sway meter fails to stay within the path. Both the maximal balance range and coordinated stability tests have been found to be reliable and sensitive to improvement following exercise intervention in older people [86]. An example of the coordinated stability test is shown in Figure 2.2.

Responses to external perturbations

Although evaluation of standing sway and reach has provided useful information regarding the interaction of musculoskeletal and sensory components of postural stability, it can only provide limited information regarding the ability to react to changing demands of a particular task. To assess this component of postural stability more closely, a number of investigations have been performed in which the subject is mechanically perturbed by applying a direct force to their body, or by tilting or translating the surface upon which they stand. These techniques are thought to provide useful information regarding how effectively the subject's sensory and motor systems respond to external stimuli, and are also capable of predicting falls.

Perhaps the simplest technique for assessing postural responses to perturbation is by applying a direct force to the subject's body, and measuring the ability of the subject to regain stability. This technique, sometimes referred to as the *postural stress test*, was first described by Wolfson et al. [87] and involves a simple pulley and weight apparatus which displaces the centre of mass behind the subject's stability limit. Performance on this task is rated on a nine-point ordinal scale which ranges from 'covert reactions' (score 9), in which the subject remains stable with little observable body displacement, and 'absent reactions' (score 0) in which the subject experiences a backwards fall. Wolfson et al. [87] reported that older nursing home-dwelling subjects scored much lower scores on the postural stress test than younger subjects, and that elderly fallers performed significantly worse on the test than nonfallers. Subsequent investigations by Chandler et al. [88] and Studenski et al. [78] achieved similar results in community-dwelling individuals with respect to fallers *versus* nonfallers; however, the Chandler et al. study reported no significant age-related differences between healthy young and older adults.

More recent investigations into responses to perturbation have utilized specialized platforms which translate in the anteroposterior and mediolateral planes or rotate coaxially with the subjects' ankle joints. The use of platform rotation as a postural perturbation was first described by Nashner [89], and was subsequently developed into the *sensory organization test*. This technique involves the modification of visual and support surface conditions; for the visual perturbation, the enclosure in which the subject is tested is rotated, while for the support surface perturbation, the platform upon which the subject stands is rotated according to

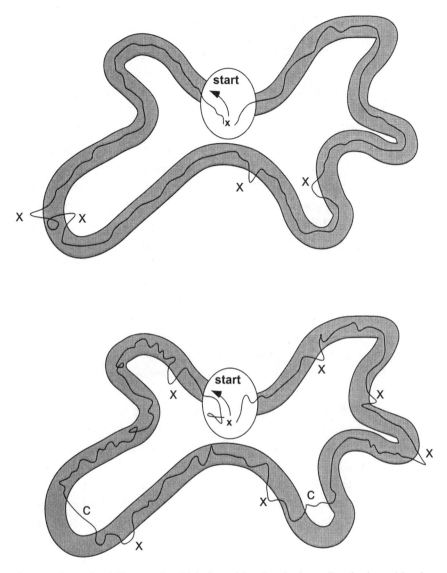

Fig. 2.2.   The coordinated stability test, in which the subject is asked to adjust body position by bending or rotating the body without moving the feet so that the pen on the end of the rod follows and remains within a convoluted track which is marked on a piece of paper attached to the top of an adjustable height table. Leaving the track scores one error point, while failing to navigate a corner scores five error points. In the top diagram, the error score is 4, while in the bottom diagram the error score is 16.

the degree of the subject's postural sway [90]. Numerous investigations utilizing this technique have reported that older subjects are less able to compensate for the altered visual and support surface conditions compared with younger adults [90–92]. This has been explained by the observation that older people have significantly slower lower-limb muscle reflex responses to rotational perturbation [90, 93, 94].

In addition to rotational perturbation, a number of authors have assessed age-related changes in response to unexpected anteroposterior and mediolateral translation of the supporting surface. Pioneering work into translational postural perturbations was undertaken by Nashner and colleagues [95–97], who established normal electromyographic responses to perturbation referred to as *muscle synergies*, in addition to describing three stereotypical postural *strategies* to compensate for different velocity perturbations. The *ankle strategy*, thought to be the most common response to standing perturbation, describes the reaction in which the subject leans forward from the ankle in response to small anteroposterior translations of the supporting surface, while the *hip strategy* involves forward trunk leaning at the level of the hip joint and occurs in response to larger perturbations. A further strategy, the *stepping strategy*, is characterized by rapid steps, hops or stumbles which occur in order to shift the base of support under the falling centre of mass when the ankle or hip strategies have failed to compensate for very large or rapid perturbations [98].

As with rotational perturbation, older people are less able to maintain stability in response to translational perturbation compared with younger adults [26, 50, 56, 99–101]. This has been explained by the observation that older people have slower muscle reflex responses to translational perturbation [38, 102], slower choice reaction time [103], and also that older people tend to utilize the hip strategy rather than the ankle strategy to maintain balance [100, 104]. Due to the increased challenge to the postural control system, translational perturbation reveals more pronounced age-related differences than unperturbed postural sway [26]. However, although differences in responses to translational perturbation have also been used to predict falls in older people [26, 56, 103], two investigations have revealed that measures of unperturbed sway may be better able to distinguish fallers from nonfallers than measures of response to perturbation [26, 56].

Recently, the *stepping strategy* has been investigated in more detail, based on the suggestion that the ability to control the centre of mass when the stability limit is moved is likely to be quite distinct from the ability to maintain balance within a stationary stability limit, and may also be a better representation of a true falling event [105]. Luchies et al. [106] assessed the responses of young and older adults when they were subjected to sudden backwards pull at the waist. Young subjects responded to the perturbation by taking a single step, while older subjects took multiple shorter steps, suggesting a decreased ability to re-establish postural stability in response to centre of mass displacement.

Similarly, McIlroy and Maki [107] assessed stepping responses in five young and nine older subjects when an anteroposterior perturbation was applied to the platform on which they stood. Although both groups of subjects performed similarly with regard to the characteristics of the first step, older subjects were twice as likely to take additional steps to maintain stability. Furthermore, the additional steps in older subjects were laterally directed in 30% of cases, suggesting the need to control for lateral instability arising after the first compensatory stepping manoeuvre.

Voluntary stepping

To avoid a fall, a three-stage response is required [103, 108]. This involves (i) perception of a postural threat, (ii) selection of an appropriate corrective response and (iii) proper response execution. To gain a single measure of this complex, multisystem response, our group has devised a test of choice reaction time that requires subjects to perform quick, correctly targeted steps in response to visual cues.

We have used this test in a recently completed study involving 510 retirement village residents aged 62–95 years [109]. These subjects stood on the choice stepping reaction time apparatus, which comprised a 0.8 m² nonslip black platform containing four white rectangular panels (32 cm × 13 cm). Two panels were situated in front of the subject (one in front of each foot), and one panel was situated on each side of the subject (adjacent to each foot). Participants were given practice trials where they were instructed to step on to the two left panels (front and side) with the left foot only and the two right panels (front and side) with the right foot only. The panels were then illuminated in a random order, and subjects were instructed to step on to the panel which was illuminated as quickly as possible but in a safe manner so as not to lose balance. Twenty trials were conducted with five trials for each of the four stepping responses. This choice stepping reaction time test is shown in Figure 2.3.

Each subject also underwent assessments of visual contrast sensitivity, lower limb proprioception, lower limb strength, simple reaction time, standing balance (postural sway) and leaning balance (maximal balance range) [55, 58, 60–62, 86, 110] and completed a questionnaire on falls in the past year.

We found that those with a history of falls had significantly increased choice reaction stepping times compared with those who reported no falls. Furthermore, ability to perform this test well was dependent upon adequate visual contrast sensitivity, lower limb extension strength, simple reaction time, and standing and leaning balance control. These measures, which have all been shown to be

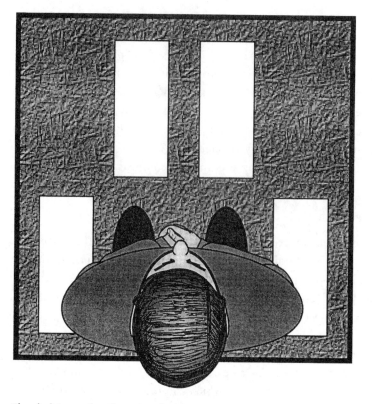

Fig. 2.3.   The choice reaction time stepping test.

important risk factors for falls in previous studies [55, 58, 60–62, 86, 110], accounted for much of the variance in choice stepping reaction time (multiple $r^2 =$ 0.42). This suggests that this new test may provide a composite measure of falls risk in older people.

Normal walking

The maintenance of balance during walking represents a considerable challenge to the postural control system. Locomotion can be regarded as consisting of four main subtasks: (i) the generation of continuous movement to progress towards a destination, (ii) maintenance of equilibrium during progression, (iii) adaptability to meet any changes in the environment, and (iv) the initiation and termination of locomotor movements [111]. Each of these tasks is heavily reliant on both the ability to generate force, and the appropriate integration of afferent input from the extremities [112, 113]. Given that ageing is associated with declines in both sensory function and muscle strength, it is clear that gait patterns will change with age and may be associated with postural instability and falling [114, 115].

A number of kinematic and kinetic studies have been undertaken to evaluate differences in gait patterns between young people and older people. The most consistent finding of these studies is that older people walk more slowly than young adults [31, 57, 116–130], which has been found to be a function of both a shorter step length [57, 116–118, 122, 123, 126, 127, 129, 131–133] and increased time spent in double limb support [57, 117, 118, 132, 133]. These temporospatial differences would appear to be a direct result of variation in self-selected walking speed, as when healthy older people and young people are instructed to walk at a specified fixed velocity, no significant differences are apparent [134]. Other gait alterations apparent in older people include reduced hip motion [117, 123, 131, 135], reduced ankle power [132, 135, 136] and range of motion [122], smaller vertical and lateral oscillations of the head [117], increased anterior pelvic tilt [132, 135] and reduced medial toe pressure [137]. Studies which have assessed foot placement have also reported that older people walk with a larger degree of out-toeing [116, 117, 132].

Age-related changes in walking patterns have generally been interpreted as indicating the adoption of a more conservative, or less destabilizing gait [111, 115, 138, 139]. However, the interpretation of gait variables in the context of postural stability is difficult, as measures of dynamic balance during gait are still being developed [140]. Winter et al. [132] have proposed an 'index of dynamic balance' to describe balance control during walking, based on the suggestion that the generation of force at the knee joint in the sagittal plane should be approximately equal to the generation of force at the hip joint if the head and trunk are to remain stable during gait. A comparison of young and older adults revealed that older subjects had a smaller index of dynamic balance and were therefore less able to control dynamically the displacement of the upper body when walking. However, the authors conceded that the functional significance of this observed difference was yet to be established.

Nevertheless, a number of investigations have revealed that certain changes in gait patterns may be predictive of falling in older people. Gait velocity, considered by some authors to be a valid measure of postural stability, has been reported to differentiate between subjects with a history of falling and those without, with fallers walking significantly slower than nonfallers [53, 54, 119, 141–144]. In addition to decreased velocity, Woolley et al. [53] also reported that fallers exhibited a significantly larger degree of out-toeing foot placement and ankle plantarflexion at heel contact. However, many of these studies have been cross-sectional, so it is possible that fallers exhibited reduced gait velocity as a result of injuries sustained from, or anxiety following, their fall. A large prospective study of 183 community-dwelling women by our group did find, however, that slow gait velocity predicts falls [57].

The functional importance and predictive value of step width measurement is unclear. In a comparative study of young and older men, Murray et al. [117] reported that step width increases significantly with normal ageing, however Gabell and Nayak [145] found no significant differences in mean step width between young and older adults. Guimaraes and Isaacs [141] and Weller et al. [146] both reported that older people with a history of falling walked with a significantly narrower step width than age-matched controls. However, these results are contradicted by similar investigations which reported no difference in step width [69] or an increased step width [147] in fallers compared with nonfallers. The lack of agreement as to whether fallers walk with a more narrow or more broad step width could be partly explained by the retrospective method used in these investigations, i.e.: it is impossible to determine whether the observed changes were a cause or a result of the fall. Furthermore, given that women tend to have narrower step widths than men [117], differences in the gender balance of the sample groups may explain some of these contradictory findings.

An alternative approach to assess gait changes associated with impaired postural control is to measure the variability of a particular gait component, rather than simply compare the mean value between fallers and nonfallers. This approach is based on the assumption that an increased variability in walking patterns is indicative of impaired motor control. Gabell and Nayak [145] evaluated gait patterns in young and older adults, and reported that although no significant differences existed between the two groups, step width and double support time values were more variable than step length and step time in both groups. This lead the authors to suggest that step length and step time are relatively stable parameters which determine the basic gait pattern, while step width and double support time may be the parameters most involved with dynamic balance control as they vary significantly from step to step.

Consistent with the suggestion that increased gait variability may represent impaired postural control, a number of studies have found that increased variability in certain gait parameters is predictive of falls in older people. A retrospective investigation by Hausdorff et al. [148] assessed gait patterns of community-dwelling older people (mean age 82 years), 18 of whom had suffered a fall in the past 5 years. Fallers walked with significantly greater variability in stride time, stance time and swing time, despite the walking speed being similar to the nonfallers. Our prospective study of 183 women [57] found that those who fell on two or more occasions in a 1-year period had a more variable cadence (stepping rate) than those who did not fall or fell on one occasion only.

Similarly, a prospective study of 75 older adults by Maki [149] reported that while mean differences in stride length, speed and double support time were not predictors of falls risk, stride-to-stride variability in these parameters were independent risk factors for falling over the 1-year follow-up period. Interestingly, this study also assessed the subjects' 'fear of falling' and reported that this was associated with reduced stride length, reduced speed and increased double support time. This finding suggests that these variables may be stabilizing adaptations related to fear of falling, rather than risk factors for falling, as previously thought. However, the interaction between fear of falling, gait alterations and falls makes it difficult to establish such a cause and effect relationship.

Tandem walking

Evaluation of an individual's ability to 'tandem walk' is a commonly used test in neurological examinations. Tandem walking is defined as walking with the feet placed in the tandem position (one foot directly in front of the other) during the double support period of the gait cycle. The constraint placed on foot position presents a further challenge to the postural control system, as the base of dynamic support is significantly reduced, leading to a reduction in mediolateral stability. This test was initially used to assess vestibular function; however, more recently it has also been adopted to assess age-related differences in lateral stability [71].

The first study to assess age-associated changes in tandem walking was conducted by Graybiel and Fregly [150], who evaluated the ability of men and women aged 13 to 50 years to walk along a range of beams of varying widths. Results revealed age to be significantly associated with beam walking performance, with older subjects less able to maintain balance on the thinner beams. More recently, a similar study by Speers et al. [71] assessed the abilities of young and older women to tandem stand and walk along beams varying in width from 2.5 cm to 15 cm. The older group performed significantly worse than the younger group, particularly on the narrowest beams. These results suggest that ageing is associated with a decreased ability to maintain balance when mediolateral stability is threatened, and that the use of beams may provide further insight into dynamic control of balance in older people.

Ability in navigating obstacles

A relatively new approach for the assessment of postural stability in older people is the evaluation of older subjects' ability to step over or avoid obstacles. The rationale behind this approach is that a large proportion of falls are related to tripping [21, 151, 152] and thus assessment of level walking may provide only limited information regarding an individual's ability to navigate around potentially hazardous environments. Furthermore, the assessment of obstacle avoidance provides further insight into the role of the 'adaptive' component of postural control [153].

The first comparative study of obstacle avoidance in young and older adults was conducted by Chen et al. [154], who assessed lower extremity kinematics when young and old subjects stepped over obstacles of 0, 25, 51 and 152 mm in height, with a 4 m approach distance. Older adults employed a more 'conservative' strategy when stepping over obstacles, exhibiting a slower 'crossing speed', shorter step length, and a smaller distance between the obstacle and the subsequent heel strike. Although none of the older subjects tripped over the obstacles, 25% stepped onto the obstacle itself, suggesting that age is associated with an increased risk of obstacle contact when walking. A subsequent study by these authors utilized 'virtual' obstacles (bands of light which fall across the path), and reported that older people require a greater response time to successfully navigate the obstacle [155].

Since the publication of the studies by Chen et al., a number of other investigators have reported similar age-associated changes in the ability to avoid obstacles, using a variety of techniques. Cao et al. [156] assessed the ability of young and older subjects to suddenly turn 90 degrees when presented with a visual stimulus along a walkway, and reported that older subjects were less able to complete the turn when provided with smaller response times. A similar study by Gilchrist [157] assessed the ability of young and older women to side step to the left or right when walking after they were presented with a visual stimulus at the end of a walkway. Fifty-eight percent of young subjects could perform the task with a single sideways step, compared with only 26% of the older subjects. In addition, older subjects' walking speed decreased significantly after the side step manoeuvre, suggesting that even when avoidance of an obstacle is successful, the older subjects were less able to incorporate the manoeuvre into their normal walking pattern.

Postural control when performing multiple tasks

A relatively recent approach to postural stability research has been to assess balance when performing cognitive tasks, based on the suggestion that dividing attention may impair postural responses to perturbation or interfere with normal gait stability. Chen et al. [158] found that older adults were more likely to step on obstacles in their path when asked to respond verbally to a visual stimulus, suggesting that older people have an increased risk of tripping when their attention is directed away from the walking task itself. Similarly, Shumway-Cook et al. [159] found that standing balance was impaired in older people when they were asked to complete a sentence and complete a visual perception matching task. In one particularly interesting recent study, Lundin-Olsson et al. [160] reported that older adults who stop walking when talking have a higher risk of falling than those who can perform both tasks simultaneously. These results suggest that falls may be more likely to occur when older adults' attention is divided between performing simple cognitive tasks and maintaining balance.

Conclusion

The maintenance of postural stability is a highly complex skill which is dependent on the coordination of a vast number of neurophysiological and biomechanical variables. Normal ageing is associated with decreased ability to maintain postural stability in standing (both bipedally and unipedally), when responding to unexpected perturbations, during normal gait and tandem gait, and when avoiding obstacles. This decrease in postural stability in older people may be explained by deficits in muscle strength, peripheral sensation, visual acuity, vestibular function and central processing of afferent inputs. Impaired postural stability, as measured by several tests of standing, leaning, stepping and walking, has consistently been shown to be a useful predictor of falls risk in older people.

REFERENCES

1 Shumway-Cook A, Woollacott M: *Motor control: theory and practical applications.* Baltimore: Williams and Wilkins, 1995.

2 Kokman E, Bossemeyer RW, Barney J, Williams WJ. Neurological manifestations of aging. *Journal of Gerontology* 1977;32(4):411–19.

3 Thornbury JM, Mistretta CM. Tactile sensitivity as a function of age. *Journal of Gerontology* 1981;36(1):34–9.

4 Kaplan FS, Nixon JE, Reitz M, Rindfleish L, Tucker J. Age-related changes in proprioception and sensation of joint position. *Acta Orthopaedica Scandinavica* 1985;56:72–4.

5 Lord SR, Ward JA. Age-associated differences in sensori-motor function and balance in community dwelling women. *Age and Ageing* 1994;23:452–60.

6 Sheldon JH. The effect of age on the control of sway. *Gerontologica Clinica* 1963;5:129–38.

7 Fitzpatrick R, Rogers DK, McClosky DI. Stable human standing with lower-limb muscle afferents providing the only sensory input. *Journal of Physiology* 1994;480:395–403.

8 Simoneau GG, Leibowitz HW, Ulbrecht JS, Tyrell RA, Cavanagh PR. The effects of visual factors and head orientation on postural steadiness in women 55 to 70 years of age. *Journal of Gerontology* 1992;47:M151–8.

9 Fitzpatrick R, McCloskey D. Proprioceptive, visual and vestibular thresholds for the perception of sway during standing in humans. *Journal of Physiology* 1994;478:173–86.

10 Shumway-Cook A, Horak F. Assessing the influence of sensory interaction on balance: suggestion from the field. *Physical Therapy* 1986;66:1548–50.

11 Lord SR, Clark RD, Webster IW. Postural stability and associated physiological factors in a population of aged persons. *Journal of Gerontology* 1991;46(3):M69–76.

12 Orma EJ. The effects of cooling the feet and closing the eyes on standing equilibrium: different patterns of standing equlibrium: in young adult men and women. *Acta Physiologica Scandinavica* 1957;38:288–97.

13 Magnusson M, Enbom H, Johansson R, Wiklund J. Significance of pressor input from the human feet in lateral postural control. *Acta Otolaryngologica* 1990;110:321–7.

14 Magnusson M, Enbom H, Johansson R, Pyykko I. Significance of pressor input from the human feet in anterior-posterior postural control. *Acta Otolaryngologica* 1990;110:182–8.

15 Romberg M. A manual of the nervous diseases of man. *Sydenham Transactions* 1853;2:396.

16 Hellbrandt FA, Braun GL. The influence of sex and age on the postural sway of man. *American Journal of Physical Anthropology* 1939; XXIV:347–60.

17 Boman K, Jalavisto E: Standing steadiness in old and young persons. *Annales Medicinae Experimentalis et Biologiae Fenniae* 1953;31:447–55.

18 Fregly AR, Graybiel A. An ataxia test battery not requiring rails. *Aerospace Medicine* 1968;39:277–82.

19 Murray M, Seirig A, Sepic S. Normal postural stability and steadiness: quantitative assessment. *Journal of Bone and Joint Surgery (Am)* 1975;57:510–16.

20 Hasselkus BR, Shambes GM. Aging and postural sway in women. *Journal of Gerontology* 1975;30(6):661–7.

21 Overstall PW, Exton-Smith AN, Imms FJ, Johnson AL. Falls in the elderly related to postural imbalance. *British Medical Journal* 1977;I:261–4.

22 Brocklehurst JC, Robertson D, James-Groom P. Clinical correlates of sway in old age: sensory modalities. *Age and Ageing* 1982;11:1–10.

23 Era P, Heikkinen E. Postural sway during standing and unexpected disturbance of balance in random samples of men of different ages. *Journal of Gerontology* 1985;40(3):287–95.

24 Ekdahl C, Jarnlo GB, Andersson SI. Standing balance in healthy subjects. *Scandinavian Journal of Rehabilitative Medicine* 1989;21:187–95.

25 Ring C, Nayak USL, Isaacs B. The effect of visual deprivation and proprioceptive change on postural sway in healthy adults. *Journal of the American Geriatrics Society* 1989;37:745–9.

26 Maki BE, Holliday PJ, Fernie GR. Aging and postural control: a comparison of spontaneous- and induced-sway balance tests. *Journal of the American Geriatrics Society* 1990;38:1–9.

27 Pyykko I, Jantti P, Aalto H. Postural control in elderly subjects. *Age and Ageing* 1990;19:215–21.

28 Peterka RJ, Black FO. Age-related changes in human posture control: sensory organization tests. *Journal of Vestibular Research* 1990;1:73–85.

29 College NR, Cantley P, Peaston I, Brash H, Lewis S, Wilson JA. Ageing and balance: the measurement of spontaneous sway by posturography. *Gerontology* 1994;40:273–8.

30 Baloh RW, Fife TD, Zwerling L, et al. Comparison of static and dynamic posturography in young and older normal people. *Journal of the American Geriatrics Society* 1994;42:405–12.

31 Okuzumi H, Tanaka A, Haishi K, Meguro K-I, Yamazaki H. Age-related changes in postural control and locomotion. *Perceptual and Motor Skills* 1995;81:991–4.

32 Baloh RW, Spain S, Socotch TM, Jacobson KM, Bell T. Posturography and balance problems in older people. *Journal of the American Geriatrics Society* 1995;43:638–44.

33 Collins JJ, DeLuca CJ, Burrows A, Lipsitz LA. Age-related changes in open-loop and closed-loop postural control mechanisms. *Experimental Brain Research* 1995; 104: 480–92.

34 McClenaghan B, Williams H, Dickerson J, Dowda M, Thombs L, Eleazer P. Spectral characteristics of ageing postural control. *Gait and Posture* 1995;3:123–31.

35 Hagemon PA. Age and gender effects on postural control measures. *Archives of Physical Medicine and Rehabilitation* 1995;76:961–5.

36 Kamen G, Patten C, Du CD, Sison S. An accelerometry-based system for the assessment of balance and postural sway. *Gerontology* 1995;44:40–5.

37 Hay L, Bard C, Fleury M, Teasdale N. Availability of visual and proprioceptive afferent messages and postural control in elderly adults. *Experimental Brain Research* 1996;108:129–39.

38 Perrin PP, Jeandel C, Perrin CA, Bene MC. Influence of visual control, conduction, and central integration on static and dynamic balance in healthy older adults. *Gerontology* 1997;43:223–31.

39 Slobounov SM, Moss SA, Slobounova ES, Newell KM. Aging and time to instability in posture. *Journal of Gerontology* 1998;53A(1):B71–8.

40 Baloh RW, Corona S, Jacobson KM, Enrietto JA, Bell T. A prospective study of posturography in normal older people. *Journal of the American Geriatrics Society* 1998;46:438–43.

41 Fernie GR, Gryfe CI, Holliday PJ, Llewellyn A. The relationship of postural sway in standing to the incidence of falls in geriatric subjects. *Age and Ageing* 1982;11:11–6.

42 Judge JO, King MB, Whipple R, Clive J, Wolfson LI. Dynamic balance in older persons: effects of reduced visual and proprioceptive input. *Journal of Gerontology* 1995;50(5):M263–70.

43 Era P, Schroll M, Ytting H, Gause-Nilsson I, Heikkinen E, Steen B. Postural balance and its sensori-motor correlates in 75-year-old men and women: a cross-national comparative study. *Journal of Gerontology* 1996;51A(2):M53–63.

44 Satariano WA, DeLorenze GN, Reed D, Schneider EL. Imbalance in an older population: an epidemiological analysis. *Journal of Ageing and Health* 1996;8(3):334–58.

45 MacLennan WJ, Timothy JI, Hall MRP. Vibration sense, proprioception and ankle reflexes in old age. *Journal of Clinical and Experimental Gerontology* 1980;2:159–71.

46 Duncan G, Wilson JA, MacLennan WJ, Lewis S. Clinical correlates of sway in elderly people living at home. *Gerontology* 1992;38:160–6.

47 Anacker SL, DiFabio RP. Influence of sensory inputs on standing balance in community-dwelling elders with a recent history of falling. *Physical Therapy* 1992;72(8):575–84.

48 Kristinsdottir EK, Jarnlo G-B, Magnusson M. Aberrations in postural control, vibration sensation and some vestibular findings in healthy 64 to 92-year-old subjects. *Scandinavian Journal of Rehabilitative Medicine* 1997;29:257–65.

49 Lichtenstein MJ, Shields SL, Shiavi RG, Burger MC. Clinical determinants of biomechanics platform measures of balance in aged women. *Journal of the American Geriatrics Society* 1988;36:996–1002.

50 Stelmach G, Phillips J, DiFabio R, Teasdale N. Age, functional postural reflexes, and voluntary sway. *Journal of Gerontology* 1989;44(4):B100–6.

51 Cohen H, Heaton LG, Congdon SL, Jenkins HA. Changes in sensory organisation test scores with age. *Age and Ageing* 1996;25:39–44.

52 Danis CG, Krebs DE, Gill-Body KM, Sahrmann S. Relationship between standing posture and stability. *Physical Therapy* 1998;78:502–17.

53 Woolley SM, Czaja SJ, Drury CG. An assessment of falls in elderly men and women. *Journal of Gerontology* 1997;52A(2):M80–7.

54 Cho C-Y, Kamen G. Detecting balance deficits in frequent fallers using clinical and quantitative evaluation tools. *Journal of the American Geriatrics Society* 1998;46:426–30.

55 Lord SR, Clark RD, Webster IW. Physiological factors associated with falls in an elderly population. *Journal of the American Geriatrics Society* 1991;39:1194–200.

56 Maki BE, Holliday PJ, Topper AK. A prospective study of postural balance and risk of falling in an ambulatory and independent elderly population. *Journal of Gerontology* 1994;49(2):M72–84.

57 Lord SR, Lloyd DG, Li SK. Sensori-motor function, gait patterns and falls in community-dwelling women. *Age and Ageing* 1996;25:292–9.

58 Lord SR, Clark RD. Simple physiological and clinical tests for the accurate prediction of falling in older people. *Gerontology* 1996;42:199–203.

59 Thapa PB, Gideon P, Brockman KG, Fought RL, Ray WA. Clinical and biomechanical measures of balance as fall predictors in ambulatory nursing home residents. *Journal of Gerontology* 1996;51A(5):M239–46.

60 Lord SR, Sambrook PN, Gilbert C, et al. Postural stability, falls and fractures in the elderly: results from the Dubbo osteoporosis epidemiology study. *Medical Journal of Australia* 1994;160:684–91.

61 Lord SR, McLean D, Stathers G. Physiological factors associated with injurious falls in older people living in the community. *Gerontology* 1992;38:338–46.

62 Lord SR, Ward JA, Williams P, Anstey K. Physiological factors associated with falls in older community-dwelling women. *Journal of the American Geriatrics Society* 1994;42:1110–17.

63 Kirby RL, Price NA, MacLeod DA. Influence of foot position on standing balance. *Journal of Biomechanics* 1987;20:423–7.

64 Goldie PA, Bach TM, Evans OM. Force platform measures for evaluating postural control: reliability and validity. *Archives of Physical Medicine and Rehabilitation* 1989;70:510–17.

65 Kollegger H, Wober C, Baumgartner C, Deecke L. Stabilizing and destabilizing effects of vision and foot position on body sway of healthy young subjects: a posturographic study. *European Neurology* 1989;29:241–5.

66 Day BL, Steiger MJ, Thompson PD, Marsden CD. Effect of vision and stance width on human body motion when standing: implications for afferent control of lateral sway. *Journal of Physiology* 1993;469:479–99.

67 Fregly AR, Smith MJ, Graybiel A. Revised normative standards of performance of men on a quantitative ataxia test battery. *Acta Otolaryngologica* 1973;75:10–16.

68 Bohannon RW, Larkin PA, Cook AC. Decrease in timed balance scores with aging. *Physical Therapy* 1984;64:1067–70.

69 Heitmann DK, Gossman MR, Shaddeau SA, Jackson JR. Balance performance and step width in noninstitutionalized, elderly, female fallers and nonfallers. *Physical Therapy* 1989;69(11):923–31.

70 Iverson BD, Gossman MR, Shaddeau SA, Turner ME. Balance performance, force produc-

tion, and activity levels in noninstitutionalized men 60 to 90 years of age. *Physical Therapy* 1990;70:348–55.

71 Speers RA, Ashton-Miller JA, Schultz AB, Alexander NB. Age differences in abilities to perform tandem stand and walk tasks of graded difficulty. *Gait and Posture* 1998;7:207–13.

72 Crosbie WJ, Nimmo MA, Banks MA, Brownlee MG, Meldrum F. Standing balance responses in two populations of elderly women: a pilot study. *Archives of Physical Medicine and Rehabilitation* 1989;70:751–4.

73 Briggs RC, Gossman MR, Birch R, Drews JE, Shaddeau SA. Balance performance among noninstitutionalized elderly women. *Physical Therapy* 1989;69:748–56.

74 Maki BE, Holliday PJ, Topper AK. Fear of falling and postural performance in the elderly. *Journal of Gerontology* 1991;46(4):M123–31.

75 Balogun JA, Akindele KA, Nihinlola JO, Mazouk DK. Age-related changes in balance performance. *Disability and Rehabilitation* 1994;16:58–62.

76 Vellas BJ, Wayne SJ, Romero L, Baumgartner RN, Rubenstein LZ, Garry PJ. One-leg balance is an important predictor of injurious falls in older persons. *Journal of the American Geriatrics Society* 1997;45:735–8.

77 Lord SR, Rogers MW, Howland A, Fitzpatrick R. Lateral stability, sensorimotor function and falls in older people. *Journal of the American Geriatrics Society* 1999;47:1077–81.

78 Studenski S, Duncan PW, Chandler J. Postural responses and effector factors in persons with unexplained falls: results and methodologic issues. *Journal of the American Geriatrics Society* 1991;39:229–34.

79 King M, Judge J, Wolfson L. Functional base of support decreases with age. *Journal of Gerontology* 1994;49(6):M258–63.

80 Duncan PW, Weiner DK, Chandler J, Studenski S. Functional reach: a new clinical measure of balance. *Journal of Gerontology* 1990;45(6):192–7.

81 Weiner DK, Duncan PW, Chandler J, Studenski SA. Functional reach: a marker of physical frailty. *Journal of the American Geriatrics Society* 1992;40:203–7.

82 Duncan PW, Studenski S, Chandler J, Prescott B. Functional reach: predictive validity in a sample of elderly male veterans. *Journal of Gerontology* 1992;47(3):M93–8.

83 Weiner DK, Bongiorni DR, Studenski SA, Duncan PW, Kochersberger GG. Does functional reach improve with rehabilitation? *Archives of Physical Medicine and Rehabilitation* 1993;74:796–800.

84 Wernick-Robinson M, Krebs DE, Giorgetti MM. Functional reach: does it really measure dynamic balance? *Archives of Physical Medicine and Rehabilitation* 1999;80:262–9.

85 Thelen DG, Wojcik LA, Schultz AB, Ashton-Miller JA, Alexander NB. Age differences in using a rapid step to regain balance during a forward fall. *Journal of Gerontology* 1997;52A(1):M8–13.

86 Lord SR, Ward JA, Williams P. The effect of exercise on dynamic stability in older women: a randomised controlled trial. *Archives of Physical Medicine and Rehabilitation* 1996;77:232–6.

87 Wolfson LI, Whipple RH, Amerman PM. Stressing the postural response: a quantitative method for testing balance. *Journal of the American Geriatrics Society* 1986;34:845–50.

88 Chandler JM, Duncan PW, Studenski SA. Balance performance on the postural stress test: comparison of young adults, healthy elderly, and fallers. *Physical Therapy* 1990;70:410–5.

89 Nashner LM. Adaptation of movement to altered environments. *Trends in Neuroscience* 1982;5:358–61.

90 Woollacott MH, Shumway-Cook A, Nashner LM. Aging and posture control: changes in sensory organization and muscular coordination. *International Journal of Ageing and Human Development* 1986;23(2):97–114.

91 Wolfson L, Whipple R, Derby CA, et al. A dynamic posturography study of balance in healthy elderly. *Neurology* 1992;42:2069–75.

92 Whipple R, Wolfson L, Derby C, Singh D, Tobin J. Altered sensory function and balance in older persons. *Journal of Gerontology* 1993;48(Special Issue): 71–6.

93 Keshner EA, Allum JHJ, Honegger F. Predictors of less stable postural responses to support surface rotations in healthy human elderly. *Journal of Vestibular Research* 1993;3:419–29.

94 Nardone A, Siliotto R, Grasso M, Schieppati M. Influence of aging on leg muscle reflex responses to stance perturbation. *Archives of Physical Medicine and Rehabilitation* 1995;76:158–65.

95 Nashner LM. Adapting reflexes controlling the human posture. *Experimental Brain Research* 1976;58:82–94.

96 Nashner LM. Fixed patterns of rapid postural responses among leg muscles during stance. *Experimental Brain Research* 1977;30:13–24.

97 Nashner LM, Woollacott M, Tuma G. Organization of rapid responses to postural and loco-motor-like perturbations of standing man. *Experimental Brain Research* 1979;36:463–76.

98 Horak FB, Shupert CL, Mirka A. Components of postural dyscontrol in the elderly: a review. *Neurobiology of Aging* 1989;10:727–38.

99 Maki BE, Holliday PJ, Fernie GR. A posture control model and balance test for the pre-diction of relative postural stability. *IEEE Transactions on Biomedical Engineering* 1987;BME34:797–809.

100 Manchester D, Woollacott M, Zedrerbauer-Hylton N, Marin O. Visual, vestibular and somatosensory contributions to balance control in the older adult. *Journal of Gerontology* 1989;44(4):M118–27.

101 Camicioli R, Panzer VP, Kaye J. Balance in the healthy elderly: posturography and clinical assessment. *Archives of Neurology* 1997;54:976–81.

102 Peterka RJ, Black FO. Age-related changes in human posture control: motor coordination tests. *Journal of Vestibular Research* 1990;1:87–96.

103 Grabiner MD, Jahnigen DW. Modeling recovery from stumbles: preliminary data on vari-able selection and classification efficacy. *Journal of the American Geriatrics Society* 1992;40:910–13.

104 Gu M-J, Schultz AB, Shepard NT, Alexander NB. Postural control in young and elderly adults when stance is perturbed: dynamics. *Journal of Biomechanics* 1996;29:319–29.

105 Maki BE, McIlroy WE. The role of limb movements in maintaining upright stance: the 'change-in-support' strategy. *Physical Therapy* 1997;77:488–507.

106 Luchies CW, Alexander NB, Schultz AB, Ashton-Miller J. Stepping responses of young and old adults to postural disturbances: kinematics. *Journal of the American Geriatrics Society* 1994;42:506–12.

107 McIlroy WE, Maki BE. Age-related changes in compensatory stepping in response to unpredictable perturbations. *Journal of Gerontology* 1996;51A(6):M289–96.

108 Stelmach GE, Worringham CJ. Sensorimotor deficits related to postural stability. Implications for falling in the elderly. *Clinics in Geriatric Medicine* 1985;1:679–94.

109 Lord SR, Matters BR, Corcoran JM, Howland AS, Fitzpatrick RC. Choice reaction time stepping: a composite measure of the risk of falling in older people. *Gait and Posture* 1999;9:S29.

110 Lord SR, Clark RD, Webster IW. Visual acuity and contrast sensitivity in relation to falls in an elderly population. *Age and Ageing* 1991;20:175–81.

111 Woollacott MH, Tang P-F. Balance control during walking in the older adult: research and its implications. *Physical Therapy* 1997;77:646–60.

112 Woollacott MH. Gait and postural control in the ageing adult. In: Bles W, Brandt T, editors. *Disorders of posture and gait.* Amsterdam: Elsevier, 1986;325–35.

113 Dietz V. Afferent and efferent control of posture and gait. In: Bles W, Brandt T, editors. *Disorders of posture and gait.* Amsterdam: Elsevier, 1986:53–68.

114 Barron RE. Disorders of gait related to the ageing nervous system. *Geriatrics* 1967;120:113–20.

115 Sudarsky L. Geriatrics: gait disorders in the elderly. *New England Journal of Medicine* 1990;322:1441–6.

116 Murray MP, Drought AB, Kory RC. Walking patterns of normal men. *Journal of Bone and Joint Surgery (Am)* 1964;46:335–60.

117 Murray MP, Kory RC, Clarkson BH. Walking patterns in healthy old men. *Journal of Gerontology* 1969;24:169–78.

118 Finley FR, Cody KA, Finizie RV. Locomotion patterns in elderly women. *Archives of Physical Medicine and Rehabilitation* 1969;50:140–6.

119 Imms FJ, Edholm OG. Studies of gait and mobility in the elderly. *Age and Ageing* 1981;10:147–56.

120 Cunningham DA, Rechnitzer PA, Pearce ME, Donner AP. Determinants of self-selected walking pace across ages 19 to 66. *Journal of Gerontology* 1982;37(5):560–4.

121 O'Brien M, Power K, Sanford S, Smith K, Wall J. Temporal gait patterns in healthy young and elderly females. *Physiotherapy Canada* 1983;35:323–6.

122 Hagemon PA, Blanke DJ. Comparison of gait of young women and elderly women. *Physical Therapy* 1986;66:1382–7.

123 Elble RJ, Thomas SS, Higgins C, Colliver J. Stride-dependent changes in gait of older people. *Journal of Neurology* 1991;238:1–5.

124 Dobbs RJ, Lubel DD, Charlett A, et al. Hypothesis: age-associated changes in gait represent, in part, a tendency towards parkinsonism. *Age and Ageing* 1992;21:221–5.

125 Dobbs RJ, Charlett A, Bowles SG, et al. Is this walk normal? *Age and Ageing* 1993;22:27–30.

126 Oberg T, Karsznia A, Oberg K. Basic gait parameters: reference data for normal subjects, 10–79 years of age. *Journal of Rehabilitation Research and Development* 1993;30:210–23.

127 Fransen M, Heussler J, Margiotta E, Edmonds J. Quantitative gait analysis: comparison of rheumatoid arthritic and non-arthritic subjects. *Australian Journal of Physiotherapy* 1994;40:191–9.

128 Buchner DM, Cress ME, Esselman PC, et al. Factors associated with changes in gait speed in older adults. *Journal of Gerontology* 1996;51A(6):M297–302.

129 Lajoie Y, Teasdale N, Bard C, Fleury M. Upright standing and gait: are there changes in attentional requirements related to normal aging? *Experimental Aging Research* 1996;22:185–98.

130 Bohannon RW. Comfortable and maximum walking speed of adults aged 20–79 years: reference values and determinants. *Age and Ageing* 1997;26:15–19.

131 Crowinshield RD, Brand RA, Johnston RC. The effects of walking velocity and age on hip kinematics and kinetics. *Clinical Orthopedics and Related Research* 1978;132:140–4.

132 Winter DA, Patla AE, Frank JS, Walt SE. Biomechanical walking patterns in the fit and healthy elderly. *Physical Therapy* 1990;70:340–7.

133 Ferrandez A-M, Pailhous J, Durup M. Slowness in elderly gait. *Experimental Aging Research* 1990;16(2):79–89.

134 Jansen EC, Vittas D, Hellberg S, Hansen J. Normal gait of young and old men and women. *Acta Orthopaedica Scandinavica* 1982;53:193–6.

135 Kerrigan DC, Todd MK, Croce UD, Lipsitz LA, Collins JJ. Biomechanical gait alterations independent of speed in the healthy elderly: evidence for specific limiting impairments. *Archives of Physical Medicine and Rehabilitation* 1998;79:317–22.

136 Judge JO, Davis RB, Ounpuu S. Step length reductions in advanced age: the role of ankle and hip kinetics. *Journal of Gerontology* 1996;51A(6):M303–12.

137 Kernozek TW, LaMott EE. Comparisons of plantar pressures between the elderly and young adults. *Gait and Posture* 1995;3:143–8.

138 Prakash C, Stern G. Neurological signs in the elderly. *Age and Ageing* 1973;2:24–7.

139 Sudarsky L, Ronthal M. Gait disorders in the elderly: assessing the risk for falls. In: Vellas B, Toupet M, Rubenstein L, et al., editors. *Falls, balance and gait disorders in the elderly.* Paris: Elsevier, 1992:117–27.

140 Winter DA. Human balance and posture control during standing and walking. *Gait and Posture* 1995;3:193–214.

141 Guimaraes RM, Isaacs B. Characteristics of the gait in old people who fall. *International Journal of Rehabilitative Medicine* 1980;2:177–80.

142 Wolfson L, Whipple R, Amerman P, Tobin JN. Gait assessment in the elderly: a gait abnormality rating scale and its relation to falls. *Journal of Gerontology* 1990;45(1):M12–19.

143 Woo J, Ho SC, Lau J, Chan SG, Yuen YK. Age-associated gait changes in the elderly: pathological or physiological ? *Neuroepidemiology* 1995;14:65–71.

144 Luukinen H, Koski K, Laippala P, Kivela S-L. Risk factors for recurrent falls in the elderly in long-term institutional care. *Public Health* 1995;109:57–65.

145 Gabell A, Nayak USL. The effect of age on variability in gait. *Journal of Gerontology* 1984;39(6):662–6.

146 Weller C, Humphrey SJE, Kirollos C, et al. Gait on a shoestring: falls and foot separation in parkinsonism. *Age and Ageing* 1992;21:242–4.

147 Gehlsen GM, Whaley MH. Falls in the elderly. Part I, gait. *Archives of Physical Medicine and Rehabilitation* 1990;71:735–8.

148 Hausdorff JM, Edelberg HK, Mitchell SL, Goldberger AL, Wei LY. Increased gait unsteadi-

ness in community-dwelling elderly fallers. *Archives of Physical Medicine and Rehabilitation* 1997;78:278–83.

149 Maki BE. Gait changes in older adults: predictors of falls or indicators of fear ? *Journal of the American Geriatrics Society* 1997;45:313–20.

150 Graybiel A, Fregly AR. A new quantitative ataxia test battery. *Acta Otolaryngologica* 1966;61:292–312.

151 Blake A, Morgan K, Bendall M, et al. Falls by elderly people at home: prevalence and associated factors. *Age and Ageing* 1988;17:365–72.

152 Campbell AJ, Borrie MJ, Spears GF, Jackson SL, Brown JS, Fitzgerald JL. Circumstances and consequences of falls experienced by a community population 70 years and over during a prospective study. *Age and Ageing* 1990;19:136–41.

153 Schultz AB, Ashton-Miller JA, Alexander NB. What leads to age and gender differences in balance maintenance and recovery ? *Muscle and Nerve* 1997;5:S60–4.

154 Chen H-C, Ashton-Miller JA, Alexander NB, Schultz AB. Stepping over obstacles: gait patterns of healthy young and old adults. *Journal of Gerontology* 1991;46(6):M196–203.

155 Chen H-C, Ashton-Miller JA, Alexander NB, Schultz AB. Effects of age and available response time on ability to step over an obstacle. *Journal of Gerontology* 1994; 49(5): M227–233.

156 Cao C, Ashton-Miller JA, Schultz AB, Alexander NB. Abilities to turn suddenly while walking: effects of age, gender, and available response time. *Journal of Gerontology* 1997;52A(2):M88–93.

157 Gilchrist LA. Age-related changes in the ability to side-step during gait. *Clinical Biomechanics* 1998;13:91–7.

158 Chen H-C, Schultz AB, Ashton-Miller JA, Giordani B, Alexander NB, Guire KE. Stepping over obstacles: dividing attention impairs performance of old more than young adults. *Journal of Gerontology* 1996;51A(3):M116–22.

159 Shumway-Cook A, Woollacott M, Kerns KA, Baldwin M. The effects of two types of cognitive tasks on postural stability in older adults with and without a history of falls. *Journal of Gerontology* 1997;52(4):M232–40.

160 Lundin-Olsson L, Nyberg L, Gustafson Y. 'Stops walking when talking' as a predictor of falls in elderly people. *Lancet* 1997;349:617.

3

Sensory and neuromuscular risk factors for falls

As discussed in Chapter 2, human balance depends on the interaction of multiple sensory, motor and integrative systems. In this chapter we review the studies which have dealt with (i) age-related changes in the sensory and motor factors that are involved in balance control and (ii) associations between these sensory and motor factors and falls in older people. Specific areas reviewed include: visual acuity, visual contrast sensitivity, visual field dependence, proprioception, tactile sensitivity, vibration sense, vestibular sense, muscle strength, neuromuscular control and reaction time.

Age-related changes in sensorimotor function

Figure 3.1 shows the physiological systems that are the primary contributors to stability. There is a growing body of evidence that indicates that functioning of these sensory, motor and integration systems declines significantly with age and that impairment in these systems is associated with falling in elderly persons. In fact, researchers have noted many people experience age-related declines in sensorimotor function, even in the absence of any documented disease. We have also found that many older people with a history of falls have no identifiable neurological or musculoskeletal disease yet perform poorly in tests of sensorimotor function. As shown in Figure 3.2, these people mostly cite trips, slips, loss of balance and muscle weakness as the causes of their falls.

Figure 3.3 shows a theoretical representation of the 'normal' age-related decline in function in a sensorimotor system that contributes to stability. The figure shows that until age 55 years there is little change in function, but beyond this age there is a progressive decline. This decline occurs in all persons but the variability in function becomes greater as age increases. If the criterion level for a loss of balance and subsequent fall is 50 units, it can be seen that persons on the lower band reach this level by age 65 whereas those toward the upper band are still above the criterion level at 80 years of age. The figure also depicts a situation in which the onset of

REACTION TIME
- simple RT
- choice RT

VESTIBULAR SENSE
- caloric testing
- rotational testing
- optical stability
- vestibulospinal reflexes

VISION
- visual acuity
- contrast sensitivity
- depth perception
- glare sensitivity
- dark adaptation

NEUROMUSCULAR CONTROL
- tapping and coordination tests

PERIPHERAL SENSATION
- tactile sensitivity
- vibration sense
- proprioception

MUSCLE STRENGTH
- hip
- knee
- ankle

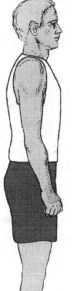

Fig. 3.1.   Systems involved in the maintenance of postural stability.

disease, such as a stroke, can rapidly change functional performance and result in performance levels below the criterion level at any age.

Vision

Many researchers have found that various visual functions including visual acuity, contrast sensitivity, glare sensitivity, dark adaptation, accommodation and depth perception decline significantly with age, especially beyond 40 years [1]. The visual function given most attention in relation to falls and falls-related injury has been visual acuity, where the published findings have been inconsistent.

In a large cross-sectional survey of eye disease with retrospective collection of falls data, Ivers et al. found that impaired visual acuity was associated with a history of recurrent falls [2]. Similarly, Nevitt et al. also found that poor visual acuity was

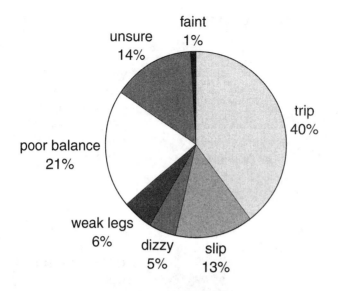

Fig. 3.2.   Causes of falls. Diagram adapted from: Lord SR, Ward JA, Williams P, Anstey KJ. An epidemiological study of falls in older community-dwelling women: the Randwick Falls and Fractures Study. *Australian Journal of Public Health* 1993;17:240–5.

a risk factor for recurrent falls in a prospective cohort study [3]. Further, they found that depth perception was similarly impaired and suggested that the association between poor visual acuity and falls may be partly indirect, as reduced visual acuity impairs depth perception. Two large prospective studies have also found that reduced visual acuity is a risk factor for hip fractures – a common consequence of falls in elderly persons [4, 5]. In one of these studies, it was noted that those with moderately good vision in one eye and good vision in the other had elevated fracture risk, indicating that poor depth perception may increase falls risk [4].

In contrast, Brocklehurst et al. [6] and Robbins et al. [7] found no associations between visual acuity and falls in age-groups above 65 years. Campbell et al. found a significant association between visual acuity and falls in a large sample of community-dwelling older people, but this association was lost when adjusting for age [8]. In one study conducted in an intermediate care facility, Tinetti et al. found an association between distant acuity loss and falls, yet in another larger study conducted in the community, such an association was not apparent although there was a significant association between near visual acuity loss and falls [9, 10].

In our studies, we have found contrast sensitivity (the detection of large visual stimuli under low-contrast conditions) to be more important than visual acuity (discrimination of fine detail) in predicting fallers [11, 12]. This finding was replicated in the Blue Mountains eye study, which compared the predictive power of a range of visual tests including visual acuity and visual field size [2]. Owen has

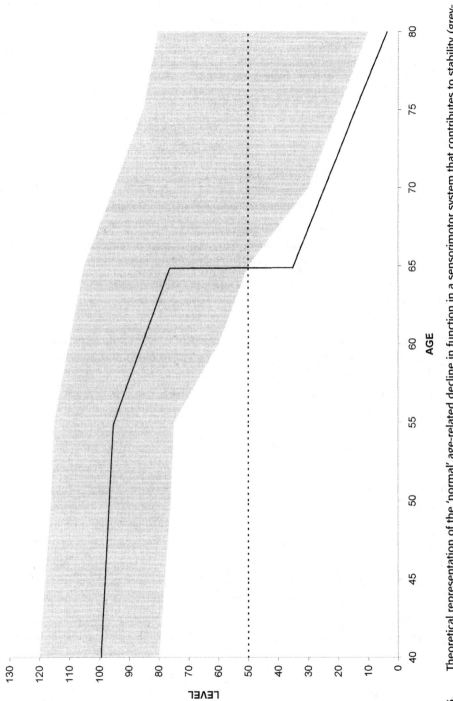

Fig. 3.3.   Theoretical representation of the 'normal' age-related decline in function in a sensorimotor system that contributes to stability (grey-shaded area represents upper and lower boundaries). The figure shows that up until age 55 years there is little change in function, but beyond this age there is a progressive decline. This decline occurs in all persons but the range in function becomes greater as age increases. The figure also depicts a situation in which the onset of disease such as a stroke (dark line) can rapidly change functional performance and result in performance levels below the criterion (dashed line) at any age.

suggested that age-related loss in contrast sensitivity, particularly to low and intermediate spatial frequencies, is likely to impair an older person's ability to detect and discriminate objects in a naturally cluttered environment [13]. As a consequence, it could be expected that an impairment in the ability to perceive edges in the environment – such as steps, gutters, tree roots and pavement cracks and misalignments could contribute to trips in older people.

Visual field dependence

In spite of the demonstrated deterioration of vision with age, it has been suggested that old people may place greater reliance on the spatial framework provided by vision in an attempt to compensate for reduced vestibular and peripheral sensation [14]. Thus in situations where minimal, ambiguous or misleading spatial information is provided by vision, body position may be wrongly determined and a fall may result. In test situations which place visual and postural cues in conflict (i.e. exposing older people to tilted or rolling visual stimuli) it has been found that older fallers are more reliant on the visual spatial framework (that is they are more field dependent) than older nonfallers [12, 15, 16].

As these studies have been undertaken in artificial situations, the findings may only partly generalize to real-world situations. The implications, however, are that tilted, moving or rolling visual stimuli, such as tilted forms and landmarks, congested pedestrian or vehicular traffic, moving vehicles, structures and shadows may contribute to falls in older people with impaired postural control.

Peripheral sensation

Scientific interest in peripheral sensation dates back to 1830 when Mueller mentioned vibration sense briefly in a textbook of physiology [17]. At the turn of the century, a number of clinicians noted that vibration sense of older persons was inferior to that of younger ones. It was not until 1928, however, that Pearson clearly demonstrated that vibration sense decreased with age [18]. Since then many investigators, using numerous vibrating stimuli, placed on various parts of the body, have consistently found age-related declines in vibration sense to all vibration frequencies greater than 50 Hz [19–33]. It has also been found that vibration sense is poorer in the lower limb compared with the upper limb at all ages and shows a greater age-related decline [21–25, 30, 32].

Scientific interest in tactile sensitivity also dates back to the nineteenth century, although there have been comparatively few studies on the effect of age on this sensory modality. Like vibration sense, most reports indicate that tactile sensitivity, as measured by aesthesiometers or by two-point discrimination, decreases significantly with age [32, 34–39] and is reduced in the lower limb compared with the upper limb [32, 35, 38, 40].

Even fewer studies have been undertaken on the effect of age on joint position sense. Laidlaw and Hamilton were the first researchers to demonstrate an age-related decline in joint position sense [41]. They found that subjects aged 17 to 35 years had lower thresholds and superior ability to detect direction of joint movements of the hip, knee and ankle than subjects aged 50 to 85 years. Since then, further studies have found significant age-related declines in position sense of the knee joint [42–45], metacarpophalangeal joint [46] and metatarsophalangeal joint [47]. However, clinical studies which have investigated whether there is a decline in joint position sense beyond 65 years of age have produced inconsistent results. This may be due at least in part to the imprecision of the tests used, which have been based on subjects' ability to identify experimenter-induced movements of body parts [6, 47, 48].

It has also been pointed out that caution should be used in assessing joint position sense when assessments are made while subjects are in the seated position [49], as is the case in all of the above studies. This is because thresholds in the ankle may be as much as 10 times lower when measured in the standing, weight-bearing position [50], where engagement of the leg muscles is greatly increased [51].

However, recent investigations assessing position sense of the ankle joint when weight bearing have also reported increased thresholds with age. For example, Thelen et al. [52] compared the ability of young and older women to detect dorsiflexion and plantarflexion movements of the foot when weightbearing on a moveable platform, and reported that the threshold for movement detection was 3–4 times larger in the older group. High detection thresholds for inversion and eversion movements of the ankle when standing either unipedally or bipedally on a rotating platform have also been found in older people [53] and in people with neuropathy [54]. Finally, Blaszczyk et al. [55] have reported that older subjects are significantly worse than young subjects in reproducing ankle joint positions when standing on a rotating platform.

It is surprising then that reduced peripheral sensation or neuropathy has been rarely mentioned as a cause of instability or falls. Robbins et al. found that lower extremity 'sensory abnormalities' were associated with falls in one of two populations studied [7] and Buchner et al. reported peripheral neuropathy to be a cause of falls in patients with Alzheimer's disease [56]. Brocklehurst et al, however, reported a significant association between impaired proprioception in the ankle and/or great toe in only one of three age-groups (75–84 years) above 65 years of age [6], whilst Nevitt et al., Wolfson et al. and Grisso et al. found no significant associations between crude measures of impaired peripheral sense and falling in their studies [3, 57, 58].

In contrast, a recent study by Richardson et al. found a strong association between electromyographically documented polyneuropathy involving the lower extremities and falls [59]. In a related study, our group has found that in both men and women, elderly subjects with diabetes performed significantly worse in tests of body sway on firm and compliant surfaces compared with the nondiabetic subjects [60]. Richardson et al. suggested that the failure to find a relationship between peripheral neuropathy and falling in previous reports may be due to the limited accuracy of clinical examinations in diagnosing neuropathy.

In all of our studies, which have been undertaken both in community and institutionalized settings, we have found that tactile sensitivity at the lateral malleolus is inferior in fallers compared with nonfallers [11, 12, 61, 62]. In a large prospective community study, we have also found that fallers demonstrate reduced vibration sense at the tibial tuberosity and impaired lower limb proprioception compared with nonfallers [62]. Impaired lower limb proprioception was also associated with multiple falls in elderly people in hostel care [11].

Thus it seems that reduced peripheral sensation is associated with falls, but that such an association only emerges when the measures of peripheral sensation are accurately and quantitatively ascertained.

Vestibular sense

The vestibular system contributes to posture by maintaining the reflex arc keeping the head and neck in the vertical position and by corrective movements elicited through the vestibulo-ocular and vestibulospinal pathways [49]. Some investigators have reported disturbed vestibular reflexes in about one-third of old people, and reduced reactivity to caloric and rotational stimulation with age beyond 60 years has been reported by a number of investigators [63, 64].

In spite of this apparent age-related decline in function, no reports have documented associations between impaired vestibular function and either instability or falls in older people. Nashner [65] found that the otoliths play no role in the initial detection of body sway, and Brocklehurst et al. [6] reported no correlation between vestibular sense as measured by response to a slow tilt and sway or falls. We also have found that vestibular function, as measured by Fukuda's vertical writing and stepping tests, or by a test of vestibulo-ocular stability is not related to stability [66, 67] or falls [62]. However, it is acknowledged that in our assessments the elderly subjects with very poor balance could not perform two of the tests, as they were incapable of walking on a treadmill or walking unsupported on the spot with the eyes closed for 1 minute.

These assessments of vestibular function have been indirect and possibly too insensitive to be able to detect subtle yet significant impairments in vestibular function. Vestibular function is less amenable to measurement or intervention than vision or peripheral sensation, and further research is required to elucidate the significance of vestibular input, and in particular otolithic functioning, to balance control.

Muscle strength

There are numerous reports of loss of isometric and dynamic muscle strength with age. In men, muscle strength appears to decrease only marginally between 20 and 40 years, but beyond 40 years declines at an accelerated pace, so that hand grip strength is reduced by 16% and leg strength by 28% in men aged 60–69 years compared with men aged 20–29 years [68–70]. In women, muscle strength appears to decline from an earlier age and at a greater rate, so that over the same age range, hand grip strength declines by 20% and leg strength by 38%. It has also been shown that muscle strength continues to decline significantly beyond the sixties in both sexes [71]. In studies that have used both men and women, it has been found that muscle strength in women is about 60–70% of that in men [68–70].

Leg extensor power (the product of force and the rate of force generation) appears to decline at an even greater rate with age than does isometric strength. In a cross-sectional study of 100 men and women aged 65–89 years, Skelton et al. [72] found a loss of isometric strength of 1–2% per annum, whereas the loss of leg extensor power was around 3.5% per annum. Increased age is also associated with a deterioration of muscle elastic behaviour and reflex potentiation [73].

Muscle weakness in the lower limbs has serious practical implications for older persons. Pearson et al. [74] found that in 14% of women aged 75 years and over living in the community the calf muscle was not able to exert sufficient force to support the body weight. This indicates that these women would be at risk of falling in situations where they place their total body weight on one leg only, i.e. when undertaking everyday activities like stepping up a stair. Vandervoort and Hayes [75] found impaired ankle plantarflexor muscle force and power in residents of geriatric care facilities who were capable of independently performing activities of daily living. They found that the ankle plantarflexor muscles in these women exhibited considerable impairment in ability to generate stabilizing torques about the ankle joint. Reduced strength is also reflected in a difficulty in rising from a chair without the use of the hands, and it has been found that an inability to undertake this task is a significant risk factor for falls in both community [3, 8] and institutional groups of older people [76].

Strength in specific lower-limb muscle groups has also been found to be inferior in fallers compared with non-fallers. In large prospective community studies, our group has found that reduced quadriceps strength increases the risk of both falls and fractures [61, 62].

Lower limb muscle weakness has also been found to be associated with falls in nursing home and hostel residents. Whipple et al. [77] and Studenski et al. [78] both compared the strength of four lower-limb muscle groups: knee extensors, knee flexors, ankle plantarflexors and ankle dorsiflexors in residents of nursing homes with and without a history of falls. Both studies found that fallers were weaker than nonfallers in all four muscle groups, with ankle muscle weakness particularly evident in the faller groups. These findings are in accord with other studies which have also found that decreased ankle dorsiflexion [61], quadriceps [79] and hip [7] strength increase the risk of falls in residents of aged-care institutions. The consistency of these findings indicates that lower limb muscle weakness is a major risk factor for falling in older people.

Reaction time

Of all the studies on age-related changes in neurological and sensorimotor systems, reaction time has possibly been studied more than any other factor. Welford [80] has summarized the findings of 21 studies on the effect of age on reaction time and found a median increase of 26% in reaction time from the twenties to the sixties. Even allowing for factors such as the amount of practice, length of preparatory interval, physical health, mode of response and level of motivation, it has been consistently found that reaction time declines with age.

In many of our studies, we have used a simple reaction time paradigm, with a simple motor response, i.e. pressing a switch, so as to emphasize the decision time component of the task. We found that in elderly community-dwelling women and elderly persons living in hostel care, increased reaction time was an independent risk factor for multiple falls [11]. Grabiner and Jahnigen [81] have also found that fallers record significantly slower reaction times than nonfallers in both simple and choice reaction time tests that involve more complicated motor responses, i.e. extending and flexing the knee. Adelsberg et al. [82] have also found that choice reaction time in those who have suffered a fracture of the lower limb is slower than in aged-matched controls.

Reaction time has been found to be independent of body sway when subjects are standing on firm surfaces after confounding effects such as age are adjusted for [66, 81]. We have noted, however, that when subjects are standing on a compliant (foam rubber) surface, reaction time is moderately associated with body sway [66, 67]. Under these conditions sway is greatly exaggerated and subjects report that they detect their body movement. Thus it seems that individuals with slow reaction time may be susceptible to falls as a result of an inability to correct postural imbalances.

Integration, interaction and summation

The above studies indicate that impairment in a number of the primary physiological systems that contribute to stability is associated with falls in older people. With such an array of inputs there is also no doubt interactions occur between the various stages in the processing of a response to a fall, i.e. sensory input and feed-forward, response selection and response execution [49, 81]. For example, much work has shown that vision can compensate for diminished peripheral input, when either experimentally induced or as a result of disease or trauma [5, 49, 83].

Our analysis suggests that while a marked impairment in just one of the physiological systems that contribute to stability is sufficient to increase the risk of falls, multiple impairments of only moderate severity are also associated with increased falls risk. For example in the case of a trip, reduced vision and slow reaction times may both be necessary for a fall to occur. Thus it seems that adequate vision and peripheral sensation allow the detection of environmental hazards, while adequate reaction time, strength and stability permit appropriate corrections to postural imbalance.

Conclusion

There is considerable evidence that the sensorimotor factors which contribute to balance control show age-related declines, and many studies have shown that over and above the effect of ageing, older people who fall demonstrate impaired functioning in these measures compared with age- and sex-matched nonfallers. Physiological systems identified as impaired in older fallers include visual functions such as contrast sensitivity and depth perception, visual field dependence, peripheral sensation, strength in the lower limb muscle groups and reaction time. The role of vestibular sense in balance and falls requires further investigation, as the tests currently used appear to be too insensitive to detect subtle deficits in vestibular function, particularly otolithic functioning.

REFERENCES

1 Pitts DG. The effects of aging on selected visual functions: dark adaptation, visual acuity, stereopsis, brightness contrast. In: Sekuler R, Kline DW, Dismukes K, editors. *Aging in human visual functions.* New York: Liss, 1982.

2 Ivers RQ, Cumming RG, Mitchell P, Attebo K. Visual impairment and falls in older adults: the Blue Mountains eye study. *Journal of the American Geriatrics* Society 1998;46:58–64.

3 Nevitt M, Cummings S, Kidd S, Black D. Risk factors for recurrent nonsyncopal falls. *Journal of the American Medical Association* 1989;261:2663–8.

4 Felson DT, Anderson JJ, Annan MT. Impaired vision and hip fracture. The Framingham study. *Journal of the American Geriatrics Society* 1989;37:495–500.

5 Diener HC, Dichgans J, Buschlbauer B, Mau H. The significance of proprioception on postural stabilization as assessed by ischaemia. *Brain Research* 1984;296: 93–9.

6 Brocklehurst JC, Robertson D, James-Groom P. Clinical correlates of sway in old age: sensory modalities. *Age and Ageing* 1982;11:1–10.

7 Robbins AS, Rubenstein LZ, Josephson KR, Schulman BL, Osterweil D, Fine G. Predictors of falls among elderly people: results of two population-based studies. *Archives of Internal Medicine* 1989;149:1628–33.

8 Campbell AJ, Borrie MJ, Spears GF. Risk factors for falls in a community-based prospective study of people 70 years and older. *Journal of Gerontology* 1989;44:M112–17.

9 Tinetti ME, Williams TF, Mayewski R. Falls risk index for elderly patients based on number of chronic disabilities. *American Journal of Medicine* 1986;80:429–34.

10 Tinetti ME, Speechley M, Ginter SF. Risk factors for falls among elderly persons living in the community. *New England Journal of Medicine* 1988;319:1701–7.

11 Lord SR, Clark RD, Webster IW. Physiological factors associated with falls in an elderly population. *Journal of the American Geriatrics Society* 1991;39:1194–200.

12 Lord SR, Sambrook PN, Gilbert C, et al. Postural stability, falls and fractures in the elderly: results from the Dubbo osteoporosis epidemiology study. *Medical Journal of Australia* 1994;160:684–91.

13 Owen DH. Maintaining posture and avoiding tripping. *Clinics in Geriatric Medicine* 1985;1:581–99.

14 Over R. Possible visual factors in falls by old people. *Gerontologist* 1966;6:212–14.

15 Lord SR, Webster IW. Visual field dependence in elderly fallers and non-fallers. *International Journal of Aging and Human Development* 1990;31:269–79.

16 Tobis JS, Reinsch S, Swanson JM, Byrd M, Scharf T. Visual perception dominance of fallers among community-dwelling older adults. *Journal of the American Geriatrics Society* 1985;33:330–3.

17 Fox JC, Klemperer WW. Vibratory sensibility: a quantitative study of its thresholds in nervous disorders. *Archives of Neurology and Psychiatry* 1942;48:622–45.

18 Pearson GHJ. Effect of age on vibratory sensibility. *Archives of Neurology and Psychiatry* 1928;20:482–96.

19 Gray RC. A quantitative study of vibration sense in normal and pernicious anaemia cases. *Minnesota Medicine* 1932;15:674–91.

20 Newman HW, Corbin KB. Quantitative determination of vibratory sensibility. *Society of Experimental Biology and Medicine* 1936;35:273–6.

21 Laidlaw RW, Hamilton MA. Thresholds of vibratory sensibility as determined by the pallesthesiometer. *Bulletin of the Neurological Institute of New York* 1937;6:494–503.

22 Cosh JA. Studies on the nature of vibration sense. *Clinical Science* 1953;12: 131–51.

23 Mirsky IA, Futterman P, Broh-Kahn RH. The quantitative measurement of vibratory percep-

tion in subjects with and without diabetes mellitus. *Journal of Laboratory and Clinical Medicine* 1953;41:221–35.

24 Steiness IB. Vibratory perception in normal subjects. *Acta Medica Scandinavica* 1957;158: 315–25.

25 Rosenberg G. Effect of age on peripheral vibratory perception. *Journal of the American Geriatrics Association* 1958;6:471–81.

26 Steinberg FU, Graber AL. The effect of age and peripheral circulation on the perception of vibration. *Archives of Physical Medicine and Rehabilitation* 1963;44:645–50.

27 Whanger AD, Wang HS. Clinical correlates of the vibratory sense in elderly psychiatric patients. *Journal of Gerontology* 1974;29:39–45.

28 Plumb CS, Meigs JW. Human vibration perception. *Archives of General Psychiatry* 1961;4: 103–6.

29 Goff GD, Rosner BS, Detre T, Kennard D. Vibration perception in normal man and medical patients. *Journal of Neurology, Neurosurgery and Psychiatry* 1965;28:503–9.

30 Perret E, Regli F. Age and the perceptual thresholds for vibratory stimuli. *European Neurology* 1970;4: 65–76.

31 Verrillo RT. Comparison of vibrotactile threshold and suprathreshold responses in men and women. *Perception and Psychophysics* 1979;26:20–4.

32 Kenshalo DR. Somesthetic sensitivity in young and elderly humans. *Journal of Gerontology* 1986;41:732–42.

33 Era P, Jokela J, Suominen H, Heikkinen E. Correlates of vibrotactile thresholds in men of different ages. *Acta Neurologica Scandinavica* 1986;74:210–17.

34 Axelrod S, Cohen LD. Senescence and embedded-figure performance in vision and touch. *Perceptual and Motor Skills* 1961;12:283–8.

35 Dyck PJ, Schultz PW, O'Brien PC. Quantification of touch-pressure sensation. *Archives of Neurology* 1972;26:465–73.

36 Gesheider GA, Bolanowski SJ, Hall KL, Hoffman KE, Verillo RT. The effects of aging on information-processing channels in the sense of touch, I. Absolute sensitivity. *Somatosensory and Motor Research* 1994;11:345–57.

37 Lord SR, Lloyd DG, Li SK. Sensori-motor function, gait patterns and falls in community-dwelling women. *Age and Ageing* 1996;25:292–9.

38 Bolton CF, Winkelmann RK, Dyck PJ. A quantitative study of Meissner's corpuscles in man. *Neurology* 1966;16:1–9.

39 Stevens JC, Choo KK. Spatial acuity of the body surface over the life span. *Somatosensory and Motor Research* 1996;13:153–66.

40 Halar EM, Hammond MC, LaCava EC, Camann C, Ward J. Sensory perception threshold measurement: an evaluation of semiobjective testing devices. *Archives of Physical Medicine and Rehabilitation* 1987;68:499–507.

41 Laidlaw RW, Hamilton NA. A study of thresholds in appreciation of passive movement among normal control subjects. *Bulletin of the Neurological Institute* 1937;6:268–73.

42 Skinner HB, Barrack RL, Cook SD. Age-related decline in proprioception. *Clinical Orthopaedics and Related Research* 1984;184:208–11.

43 Kaplan FS, Nixon JE, Reitz M, Rindfleish L, Tucker J. Age-related changes in proprioception and sensation of joint position. *Acta Orthopaedica Scandinavica* 1985;56:72–4.

44 Petrella RJ, Lattanzio PJ, Nelson MG. Effect of age and activity on knee joint proprioception. *American Journal of Physical Medicine and Rehabilitation* 1997;76:235–41.

45 Hurley MV, Rees J, Newham DJ. Quadriceps function, proprioceptive acuity and functional performance in healthy young, middle-aged and elderly subjects. *Age and Ageing* 1998;27:55–62.

46 Kokmen E, Bossemeyer RW, Williams WJ. Quantitative evaluation of joint motion sensation in an aging population. *Journal of Gerontology* 1978;33:62–7.

47 MacLennan WJ, Timothy JI, Hall MRP. Vibration sense, proprioception and ankle reflexes in old age. *Journal of Clinical and Experimental Gerontology* 1980;2:159–71.

48 Howell TH. Senile deterioration of the central nervous system. *British Medical Journal* 1949;i:56–8.

49 Stelmach GE, Worringham CJ. Sensorimotor deficits related to postural stability. Implications for falling in the elderly. *Clinics in Geriatric Medicine* 1985;1:679–94.

50 Gurfinkel VS, Lipshits MI, Popov KE. Thresholds for kinesthetic sensation in the vertical position. *Human Physiology* 1982;8:439–45.

51 Refshauge KM, Fitzpatrick RC. Perception of movement at the human ankle: effects of leg position. *Journal of Physiology* 1995;488:243–8.

52 Thelen DG, Brockmiller C, Ashton-Miller JA, Schultz AB, Alexander NB. Thresholds for sensing foot dorsi- and plantarflexion during upright stance: effects of age and velocity. *Journal of Gerontology* 1998;53:M33–8.

53 Gilsing MG, VandenBosch CG, Lee SG, et al. Association of age with the threshold for detecting ankle inversion and eversion in upright stance. *Age and Ageing* 1995;24:58–66.

54 VandenBosch C, Gilsing M, Lee S-G, Richardson J, Ashton-Miller J. Peripheral neuropathy effect on ankle inversion and eversion detection thresholds. *Archives of Physical Medicine and Rehabilitation* 1995;76:850–6.

55 Blaszczyk JW, Hansen PD, Lowe DL. Accuracy of passive ankle joint positioning during quiet stance in young and elderly subjects. *Gait and Posture* 1993;1:211–15.

56 Buchner DM, Larson EB. Falls and fractures in patients with Alzheimer-type dementia. *Journal of the American Medical Association* 1987;257:1492–5.

57 Wolfson L, Judge J, Whipple R, King M. Strength is a major factor in balance, gait, and the occurrence of falls. *Journal of Gerontology* 1995;50:S64–7.

58 Grisso JA, Kelsey JL, Strom BL, Chiu GY, Maislin G, O'Brien RN. Risk factors for falls as a cause of hip fracture in women. *New England Journal of Medicine* 1991;324:1321–6.

59 Richardson J, Ching C, Hurvitz E. The relationship between electromyographically documented peripheral neuropathy and falls. *Journal of the American Geriatrics Society* 1992;40:1008–12.

60 Lord SR, Caplan GA, Colagiuri R, Ward JA. Sensori-motor function in older persons with diabetes. *Diabetic Medicine* 1993;10:614–18.

61 Lord SR, McLean D, Stathers G. Physiological factors associated with injurious falls in older people living in the community. *Gerontology* 1992;38:338–46.

62 Lord SR, Ward JA, Williams P, Anstey K. Physiological factors associated with falls in older community-dwelling women. *Journal of the American Geriatrics Society* 1994;42:1110–17.

63 Karlsen EA, Hassanein RM, Goetzinger CP. The effects of age, sex, hearing loss and water temperature on caloric nystagmus. *The Laryngoscope* 1981;91:620–7.

64 Ghosh P. Aging and auditory vestibular response. *Ear, Nose and Throat Journal* 1985;64:264–6.

65 Nashner LM. A model describing vestibular detection of body sway motion. *Acta Otolaryngologica* 1971;72:429–36.

66 Lord SR, Clark RD, Webster IW. Postural stability and associated physiological factors in a population of aged persons. *Journal of Gerontology* 1991;46:M69–76.

67 Lord SR, Ward JA. Age-associated differences in sensori-motor function and balance in community dwelling women. *Age and Ageing* 1994;23:452–60.

68 Petrovsky JS, Burse RL, Lind AR. Comparison of physiological responses of men and women to isometric exercise. *Journal of Applied Physiology* 1975;38:863–8.

69 Murray MP, Gardner GM, Mollinger LA, Sepic SB. Strength of isometric and isokinetic contractions. Knee muscles of men aged 20 to 86. *Physical Therapy* 1980;60:412–19.

70 Murray MP, Duthie EH, Gambert SR, Sepic SB, Mollinger LA. Age-related differences in knee muscle strength in normal women. *Journal of Gerontology* 1985;40:275–80.

71 MacLennan WJ, Hall MRP, Timothy JI, Robinson M. Is weakness in old age due to muscle wasting ? *Age and Ageing* 1980;9:188–92.

72 Skelton DA, Greig CA, Davies JM, Young A. Strength, power and related functional ability of healthy people aged 65–89 years. *Age and Ageing* 1994;23:371–7.

73 Bosco C, Komi PV: Influence of aging on the mechanical behaviour of leg extensor muscles. *European Journal of Applied Physiology* 1980;45:209–19.

74 Pearson MB, Bassey EJ, Bendall MJ. Muscle strength and anthropometric indices in elderly men and women. *Age and Ageing* 1985;14:49–54.

75 Vandervoort AA, Hayes KC. Plantarflexor muscle function in young and elderly women. *European Journal of Applied Physiology* 1989;58:389–94.

76 Lipsitz LA, Jonsson PV, Kelley MM, Koestner JS. Causes and correlates of recurrent falls in ambulatory frail elderly. *Journal of Gerontology* 1991;46:M114–22.

77 Whipple RH, Wolfson LI, Amerman PM. The relationship of knee and ankle weakness to falls in nursing home residents: an isokinetic study. *Journal of the American Geriatrics Society* 1987;35:13–20.

78 Studenski, S, Duncan PW, Chandler J. Postural responses and effector factors in persons with unexplained falls: results and methodologic issues. *Journal of the American Geriatrics Society* 1991;39:229–34.

79 Luukinen H, Koski K, Laippala P, Kivela S-L. Risk factors for recurrent falls in the elderly in long-term institutional care. *Public Health* 1995;109:57–65.

80 Welford AT. Motor performance. In: Birren JE, Schiae KW, editors. *Handbook of the psychology of aging.* New York: Van Nostrand Reinhold, 1977.

81 Grabiner MD, Jahnigen DW. Modeling recovery from stumbles: preliminary data on variable selection and classification efficacy. *Journal of the American Geriatrics Society* 1992;40:910–13.

82 Adelsberg S, Pitman M, Alexander H. Lower extremity fractures: relationship to reaction time and coordination time. *Archives of Physical Medicine and Rehabilitation* 1989;70:737–9.

83 Fernie GR, Eng P, Holliday PJ. Postural sway in amputees and normal subjects. *Journal of Bone and Joint Surgery (Am)* 1978;60:895–8.

Medical risk factors for falls

It has long been recognized that frail, older people with multiple chronic illnesses experience higher rates of falls than active, healthy older people [1]. This observation suggests that rather than being a nonspecific accompaniment of ageing, many falls may occur as a result of clinically identifiable causes. Thus, differentiating the relative contribution of pre-existing disease to risk of falling is an important component of a falls prevention programme, as it enables clinicians involved in the management of older people to determine when it is appropriate to intervene medically. In this chapter, we discuss the contribution of common medical conditions (including neurological problems, cardiovascular problems, visual problems, lower extremity problems, urinary incontinence and psychological and cognitive problems) to risk of falling in older people.

Neurological problems

Stroke

Cerebrovascular accidents are common in older people, and have been associated with a two to sixfold increased risk of falling by a number of prospective investigations [2–8]. Following a stroke, many people have an inability to generate sufficient amounts of force in lower limb musculature, or to coordinate the actions of different muscle groups [9]. This may result in a decreased ability to maintain the leg extended during the stance phase of walking and decreased foot clearance during the swing phase which may result in tripping [10]. People with impaired gait following a stroke may also have difficulty adapting to challenging environments (e.g. uneven ground, obstacles).

In addition, brainstem and cerebellar strokes may cause damage to areas in the brain closely associated with balance, while sensory and visual inattention when recovering from a stroke may produce a tendency to bump into environmental hazards. Parietal lobe damage may impair the planning and execution of locomotor activities, and in cases where the frontal lobes are damaged, there is the possibility that judgement may be affected, causing the older person to take risks when navigating obstacles in the environment [10].

Parkinson's disease

Parkinson's disease is characterized by bradykinesia, tremor and muscular rigidity, and is known to affect approximately 2% of people over the age of 65 years [11]. Older people with Parkinson's disease often exhibit a flexed posture of both the trunk and limbs, and impaired postural equilibrium. The characteristic gait of the parkinsonian patient exhibits short, shuffling steps, lack of arm swing, loss of trunk movements, decreased foot clearance, and festination (fast, short steps) [12]. These changes, while not associated with increased sway when standing [13–15], are associated with impaired responses to external perturbations [16], and increased variability in stride length when walking [17–20].

Due to their rigid posture, gait, and impaired ability to respond to external perturbations, many older people with Parkinson's disease suffer from frequent falls [21–23]. These falls may result from episodes of 'freezing', in which the older person attempts to overcome an inability to initiate movement and subsequently loses balance, or from muscle shortening as a result of decreased levels of activity. Paulson et al. [21] reported that 53% of 211 subjects with Parkinson's disease suffered from frequent falls, while a study of 100 subjects with idiopathic Parkinson's disease by Koller et al. [22] reported that 38% had experienced falls, with 13% falling more than once per week. Parkinson's disease has also been found to be a strong independent risk factor for falling in epidemiological studies, in both institutionalized [24] and community-dwelling [3, 4, 25, 26] older people.

Myelopathy

Degenerative changes in the cervical spine (often referred to as cervical spondylosis) are a common finding in older people. With advancing age, the spinal canal in the cervical region of the spine becomes increasingly narrow due to ligamentous hypertrophy, intervertebral disc herniation and formation of osteophytes on cervical vertebral processes. The narrowing of the spinal canal may lead to mechanical spinal cord impingement and associated postural dysfunction referred to as myelopathy [27]. Myelopathy is commonly associated with subjective reports of clumsiness, difficulty climbing stairs and experiences of the legs 'giving way', while objective findings include standing imbalance and ataxic gait. These changes have been suggested to be associated with falls; however, no studies have reported myelopathy to be a prospective risk factor in a large sample of older people. Nevertheless, it has been suggested that myelopathy may be under-diagnosed by clinicians, and as such, may be a more common cause of falls than is generally recognized [28].

Cerebellar disorders

The vestibulocerebellum and spinocerebellum regions of the brain are of particular importance to the maintenance of postural stability. Lesions in these regions as a result of alcoholism, degeneration, ischaemia or haemorrhage have been shown to increase sway when standing [29–32]. Cerebellar lesions may also affect gait patterns by altering normal limb kinematics and interlimb coordination. Older people with cerebellar disorders tend to have trunk instability, a wide-based gait and irregular step lengths [33]. Although few authors have reported cerebellar dysfunction to be a risk factor for falls *per se* [1, 34], two of the characteristic gait variables associated with these syndromes – wide-based gait [35, 36] and irregular step lengths [37–39] – have been found to increase the risk of falling.

Vestibular pathology

Although it is well recognized that maintaining postural stability relies on the integration of visual, somatosensory and vestibular inputs, the role of the vestibular system in falls in older people still remains obscure, as do the relative contributions of the otoliths and semicircular canals which comprise the vestibular apparatus. However, the presence of severe vestibular pathology (such as Menière's disease) produces obvious impairments in posture and gait which may place the older person at an increased risk of recurrent falls.

Vestibular pathology is one of the most common causes of persistent and recurrent symptoms of dizziness in older people [40], and is classically characterized by marked postural instability when standing and a broad-based, staggering gait pattern with unsteady turns [41]. However, in cases of long-term total vestibular loss, gait may appear normal and deficits will only become apparent when the subject stands in the tandem position with eyes closed (the 'sharpened Romberg' position). This suggests that visual and somatosensory inputs may be able to compensate for absence of vestibular input, and that vestibular loss may only produce overt postural instability if vision and peripheral sensation are also impaired.

Due to the complexity of the interaction between these three systems, it has been difficult to ascertain the significance of vestibular dysfunction for falls in older people. As outlined in Chapter 3, we have not found the vestibular stepping test, the vestibular optical stability test or the vertical writing test to be strong predictors of falls in our prospective studies [42, 43]. However, the vertical writing test did predict variability in gait patterns in our study of 183 community-dwelling women [37], and performance in tests of dependence on visual-field cues was significantly worse in subjects with a history of falls compared with nonfallers [44].

Although vestibular function tests may not be strong predictors of falls, vestibular dysfunction should be considered a significant differential diagnosis in patients who have recurrent unexpected falls without loss of consciousness, paresis, sensory loss, or cerebellar deficits [45]. A recent prospective study of 50 older people complaining of dizziness found that 18% had a previously undiagnosed vestibular pathology [46], suggesting that investigation of vestibular function may explain many apparently 'idiopathic' recurrent falls.

Peripheral neuropathy

The normal ageing process is associated with reduced peripheral sensation, and numerous prospective investigations into falls in older people have found that subjects who experienced falls performed worse in tests of lower limb proprioception [42, 47–49], vibration sense [50–52] and tactile sensitivity [37, 48]. In addition to normal ageing, peripheral neuropathy can result from a wide range of causes, including diabetes mellitus, alcohol abuse, vitamin B12 deficiency, chemotherapy, and overdose of pyridoxine or nitric oxide [53]. Of these, the most common cause of peripheral neuropathy is diabetes mellitus. Peripheral nerve damage occurs in up to 25% of patients with diabetes mellitus after 10 years of being diagnosed with the disease, and in up to 50% of patients after 20 years disease duration [54]. People with diabetic neuropathy have impaired standing stability compared with age-matched controls [55–57] and perform worse in tests of foot position sense [58, 59]. The presence of diabetic neuropathy has also been found to increase the risk of fall-related injury by up to 15 times [60–62]. The available evidence therefore suggests that peripheral neuropathy, by affecting the ability of an older person to perceive the orientation and movements of the limbs, is a significant risk factor for falls and fall-related injuries.

Cardiovascular problems resulting in neural failure of postural control

Orthostatic hypotension

Orthostatic hypotension, also known as *postural hypotension*, refers to the drop in blood pressure which occurs when transferring from a supine to a standing position. Two broad categories are recognized. *Asymptomatic* orthostatic hypotension is a drop in systolic pressure of 20 mmHg or diastolic pressure of 10 mmHg or more at 1–5 minutes after moving from the supine to the standing position without symptoms. *Symptomatic* orthostatic hypotension results in subjects reporting dizziness, lightheadedness or faintness to the extent that the procedure of measuring standing blood pressure must be aborted [63, 64].

The reported prevalence of orthostatic hypotension in older people ranges from 6% to 33% [65–75]. This large variation can be attributed to variations in the sample assessed, the technique of blood pressure measurement performed, and the definitions employed [63, 67, 70]. A major limitation of many of these studies is that they have not excluded subjects with chronic diseases or those taking medications known to cause orthostatic hypotension. Thus, the prevalence reported may overestimate the true prevalence in healthy, community-dwelling older people. When confounding variables are adjusted for, prevalence of orthostatic hypotension in community-dwelling older people is approximately 6% [75, 76]. These results suggest that orthostatic hypotension is relatively uncommon in community-dwelling healthy older people, and tends to be associated with pre-existing disease or use of medications which have antihypertensive effects.

The most common cause of orthostatic hypotension is the failure of the autonomic nervous system to react to the body's change in posture [77, 78]. However, numerous diseases have also been found to be associated with an increased risk of developing orthostatic hypotension, including heart failure, diabetes mellitus, Parkinson's disease, stroke, dementia and depression [76, 79, 80]. Drugs known to induce orthostatic hypotension include antihypertensives, anti-Parkinsonian drugs, antidepressants, antipsychotics and diuretics [81, 82]. After controlling for disease states and medication use, there does not appear to be a significant association with advancing age [76], nor are there consistent gender differences. However, given the increased prevalence of both disease and medication risk factors with advancing age, it is not surprising that prevalence of orthostatic hypotension has been found to increase with age when these variables are not controlled for [63, 66, 83].

The association between orthostatic hypotension and falls dates back to Sheldon's 1960 study, in which 4% of 500 falls in 202 older people were attributed to 'abnormal blood pressure homeostasis' [84]. Numerous retrospective studies have since provided further evidence to support a relationship between orthostatic hypotension and falls [47, 85–88]. Brocklehurst et al. have also suggested that 20% of hospital admissions for hip fracture could be attributed to hypotension-related loss of consciousness [89]. In contrast to these findings, a post-fall assessment study conducted by Kirshen et al. [90] reported that *none* of the falls reported in two residential care facilities could be attributed to orthostatic hypotension, and Salgado et al. [5] did not find any difference in prevalence of orthostatic hypotension in older people who had and had not fallen while in hospital.

The validity of the results of these studies is limited by the retrospective design employed, and no prospective investigations have reported orthostatic hypotension as a strong risk factor for falls. Studies conducted by our research group have failed to show orthostatic hypotension to be a strong risk factor for falling. A 12-month prospective study of 81 hostel residents revealed that antihypertensive medications were not a risk factor for falls, and none of the subjects exhibited orthostatic hypotension when blood pressure was measured in supine and standing positions [91]. Similarly, investigations of 414 community-dwelling older women aged 65 to 99 years [92] and 81 hostel-dwelling older people [93] found that orthostatic hypotension was not a risk factor for falling in the 12-month follow-up period. Similar results were reported in a recent prospective study by Liu et al. [94], who found no association between falls and orthostatic hypotension or use of diuretic medications.

Delineating the role of orthostatic hypotension in falls is inherently difficult due

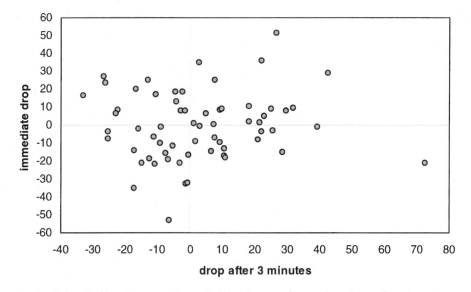

Fig. 4.1.   Postural drop in blood pressure immediately after standing and 3 minutes later in 67
older people.

to (i) differences in the way blood pressure has been measured; (ii) the normal variations in blood pressure from day to day and following meals; (iii) the weak correlation between subjective reporting of dizziness and objective measures of blood
pressure; and (iv) the fact that even transient illness may cause a drop in blood pressure. Differences in blood pressure protocols are a significant concern when inter-
preting the results of studies on orthostatic hypotension and falls. While standard
definitions and measurement techniques for orthostatic hypotension have now
been documented [95], earlier investigations have utilized different protocols
which may not produce equivalent values. In particular, the time period between
supine measurement and standing measurement has varied from 1 [76] to 5
minutes [96]. Figure 4.1 shows a plot of postural drop in blood pressure in 67 older
people, measured with a finger blood pressure cuff immediately after standing and
then 3 minutes later. As can be seen from the graph, there is little association
between the two measures. Clearly, values obtained using different measurement
protocols cannot be directly compared.

Blood pressure has been found to vary considerably both during the day and
from one day to the next in older people [97] and, as such, orthostatic hypotension
measurement has been found to have poor reproducibility [98]. One major cause
of this variation is blood pressure reduction following consumption of food (post-
prandial hypotension) [99, 100], which commonly occurs in active and well older
people [101]. There is only weak evidence that the drop in blood pressure following consumption of food could be associated with falling. Two retrospective studies

[88, 102] have reported that post-prandial hypotension is more marked in older people with a history of falling, although no prospective evidence exists. These results suggest that assessing the contribution of orthostatic hypotension to risk of falling is a 'hit and miss' affair, as the effects are transient, and the results of falls investigations could vary considerably depending on when blood pressure measurements are performed.

A final limitation of the literature pertaining to orthostatic hypotension and falls relates to the fact that only weak correlations have been reported between objectively measured orthostatic hypotension and subjective reports of dizziness [76, 85, 103–105]. This explains why orthostatic symptoms can exist without the presence of objectively measured orthostatic hypotension [96] and why individuals with orthostatic hypotension do not always exhibit symptoms [104]. Interestingly, a cross-sectional study by Ensrud et al. [104] reported that only 23% of subjects diagnosed with orthostatic hypotension experienced feelings of dizziness. In addition, although measurement of orthostatic hypotension was only weakly associated with falls, self-reported 'dizziness' was significantly associated with increased falls risk. This suggests that symptoms of dizziness, rather than objective measurement of orthostatic hypotension, may be a more accurate predictor of falls, and that reports of dizziness should not be interpreted as diagnostic of orthostatic hypotension.

The confusion in the literature pertaining to dizziness in older people was the subject of a recent editorial in the *Journal of the American Geriatrics Society* [106]. The authors suggested that, due to the variety of ways causes of dizziness have been classified in the literature, the results of various studies are analogous to the story of the blind men and the elephant. In this story, three blind men each feel a different part of the elephant's body, and each observation provides accurate but biased information as to what the elephant is like.

Drop attacks

The term 'drop attack' was first used by Sheldon [84], and refers to a sudden, unexpected fall to the ground preceded by turning of the head or tilting of the neck. The victim of a drop attack does not experience any loss of consciousness; however, there is often a transient loss of strength in the legs and trunk [107]. Since this early description, the term 'drop attack' has been variably applied to a range of neurological phenomena associated with falls, and in common usage is a blanket term covering unexpected falls without a loss of consciousness.

The causative mechanism of a drop attack is still poorly understood, and indeed in many cases no cause can be identified [108]. Sheldon's original description suggested that the 'sudden loss of postural alertness' associated with the condition could be attributed to brainstem dysfunction [84], while more recent studies have implicated vertebral–basilar artery insufficiency [109–113], structural lesions of the cervical spine [114, 115], and carotid sinus hypersensitivity [116–119]. While drop attacks can occur in otherwise healthy individuals, they are also commonly associated with neurological conditions including Menière's disease [120, 121] and epilepsy [122, 123].

Drop attacks have been reported as the cause of between 2% and 25 % of falls [84, 85, 89, 124–126], but the definition of a drop attack and the population studied varies considerably in the literature. Sheldon's study attributed 25% of the 500 falls in community-dwelling women to a drop attack [84], while Clark [124], using the same definition, found that 16% of 431 fall-related hip fractures in women could be attributed to drop attacks, with an increasing prevalence of drop attacks with advancing age. Campbell et al. [85] also noted an increased prevalence of drop attacks with advancing age, but reported a smaller overall prevalence of 16% of all falls. An investigation of fall-related hip fractures in hospital reported that 20% of the 348 falls were due to drop attacks; however, the definition of a drop attack also included 'giddiness' and vertigo [89]. These results would seem to suggest that drop attacks are a common cause of falls in older people.

More recent investigations have tended to focus on developing multiple sensory and motor risk factors for falls, and as a result, drop attacks have not received the same focus as earlier studies. Nevertheless, it is possible that carotid sinus hypersensitivity, often cited as a cause of drop attacks, may be responsible for some proportion of the 'unexplained' falls in these investigations. A retrospective study of 200 fallers admitted to a hospital emergency department found that 30% were unable to recall a reason for their fall, and of these, 73% exhibited carotid sinus hypersensitivity [127]. Similarly, Richardson et al. [128] found that 23% of older people presenting to an accident and emergency department with 'unexplained' or 'recurrent' falls exhibited carotid sinus hypersensitivity. However, it is also possible that older people with poor vision, reduced sensation and slowed reaction time may fall as a result of a trip or slip, but be unaware as to why they fell, and subsequently be diagnosed with a drop attack.

In summary, it would appear that drop attacks may be responsible for a number of falls that cannot to be explained by multiple sensory and motor risk factor assessments. However, the evidence for drop attacks as a cause of falls is primarily retrospective, and is marred by the use of inconsistent definitions across the literature. Furthermore, given that carotid sinus hypersensitivity is common in older people [129], a strong causal relationship with falling has been difficult to establish. It could therefore be argued that the prevalence of drop attacks may be overestimated, and it is possible that if thorough sensorimotor assessments were conducted on older people diagnosed with a drop attack, factors such as reaction time, poor vision, increased sway and visual field dependence could explain a considerable number of these falls. Nevertheless, there would appear to be some merit in the suggestion that older people with recurrent, unexplained falls be assessed for carotid sinus hypersensitivity, as it is amenable to treatment with cardiac pacemakers. However, carotid sinus massage is potentially harmful and must be carefully performed by cardiologists only in very select circumstances [118].

Syncope

One of the 'grey' areas in the falls literature is the role of loss of consciousness. A myriad of cardiac, haemodynamic, metabolic and psychiatric factors may cause a loss of consciousness, and invariably this will cause the older person to fall. However, falls researchers have approached the role of loss of consciousness in different ways; some have differentiated 'multifactorial' falls from those caused by an obvious loss of consciousness, while others have included these types of falls in their analysis. Consequently, the literature pertaining to falls and loss of consciousness is somewhat perplexing.

Syncope can be defined as a temporary loss of consciousness with spontaneous recovery, and occurs when there is a transient decrease in cerebral blood flow. This can be caused by several cardiac and haemodynamic factors, including orthostatic hypotension, vasovagal attacks, transient ischaemic attacks, carotid sinus hypersensitivity, cardiac arrhythmia, and aortic stenosis. However, the cause of syncope cannot be determined in up to 50% of cases [130, 131]. Post-prandial hypotension is also often cited as a cause of syncope in older people, although it would appear that the drop in blood pressure following a meal will only cause the subject to lose consciousness in the presence of antihypertensive medication usage [132], Parkinson's disease [133] or autonomic dysfunction [134]. A recent study of 33 patients with 'unexplained' syncope reported that 36% could be attributed to vasovagal attacks, 15% to cardiac arrhythmia, 9% to antihypertensive medications, 6% to orthostatic hypotension, and in one case, hyperventilation due to anxiety [135]. The relationship between cardiovascular dysfunction and syncope has also been highlighted in a recent study by Lawson et al. [136], who reported that the presence of syncope in patients who report severe dizziness is an accurate predictor of an eventual cardiovascular diagnosis.

The significance of syncope in elderly falls, however, is very difficult to determine, as loss of consciousness is often associated with amnesia, making retrospective assessments difficult. In addition, many studies consider falls and syncope to be two separate diagnoses with two separate sets of aetiologies, rather than viewing syncope as a precursor of falling [137]. This may explain why syncope has been reported as the cause of only 3% of falls in both nursing home [47, 87] and community-dwelling [34, 84, 89] populations. However, there is some evidence that falls caused by syncope may be more likely to cause serious injury than falls without a loss of consciousness [138], presumably because the older person is unable to make any postural adjustments to minimize the impact of the fall.

The major limitation of the literature on syncope and falls, however, is the confusion caused by the interchangeable use of the terms syncope and drop attack, in addition to their 'shared' suspected aetiologies (orthostatic hypotension, postprandial hypotension, carotid sinus hypersensitivity, etc.). For example, some studies record syncope as a *cause* of drop attacks [119], and both syncope and drop attacks may be caused by carotid sinus hypersensitivity. This confusing use of terminology and complex causal inter-relationships may be primarily responsible for the limited understanding of the significance of syncope in falls in older people.

Visual problems

With ageing, the eye undergoes numerous physiological changes associated with the inevitable decline in visual acuity with advancing age [139, 140]. As outlined in Chapter 3, many authors have reported visual impairment, including poor contrast sensitivity [141, 142], poor visual acuity [93, 143], impaired depth perception [4] and self-reported poor vision [144] to be a strong risk factor for falls in older people. In addition to normal age-related visual decline, older people are also particularly susceptible to developing visual deficits from common eye pathologies such as cataracts, macular degeneration or glaucoma. However, the contribution of these pathologies to risk of falling is difficult to ascertain, as many studies use visual acuity tests as measures of visual impairment rather than relying on previous diagnoses of eye disease. Nevertheless, although there is relatively little evidence associating falls risk with specific diagnoses, it is clear that eye diseases exacerbate age-related visual loss and thereby increase falls risk.

Cataracts

The term 'cataract' refers to an increase in the opacity of the lens, leading to smoky, cloudy or hazy vision. Although cataracts are predominantly a disease of old age, the changes in the molecular structure of the lens due to the ageing process itself do not fully explain the production of cataracts. There is a general consensus that cataracts form as a result of complex biochemical reactions which eventually lead to oxidation of the lens, membrane breakdown and eventual opacity, while ageing increases the susceptibility of the lens to the detrimental effects of these oxidative agents [145]. Cataracts affect approximately 16% of people over the age of 65 [146], and are a common cause of impaired vision in older people.

A small number of studies have found cataracts to be associated with increased risk of falling. A 10-year prospective study of 2633 older people by Felson et al. [147] reported that 18% of hip fractures in the follow-up period were associated with visual impairment, with cataracts being the most common cause. Sim. Jack et al. [143] reported that older people admitted to hospital for a fall were likely to have visual impairment than those admitted for other reasons, and 37% of these patients had cataracts. More recently, cataracts were found to be an independent risk factor for falls in 465 community-dwelling older people [7], while a large cross-sectional study of 3299 people over the age of 49 years in Australia reported that the presence of cataracts was significantly associated with increased risk of suffering two or more falls in the previous 12 months [148]. These results indicate that cataracts are associated with an increased risk of falling in older people.

Macular degeneration

Several disorders can lead to degenerative lesions of the macular region of the retina. Age-related macular degeneration is the most common and serious form, affecting approximately 9% of older people aged over 65 years [146], and up to 19% of people over 85 years of age [149]. Age-related macular degeneration is recognized as the leading cause of blindness among older people in industrialized countries [150]. Despite the recognition of macular degeneration as a common and serious eye disease, few studies have assessed the role of macular degeneration as a risk factor for falls. The Blue Mountains eye study in Australia found that the presence of macular degeneration was not a statistically significant risk factor for falls in their sample of 3299 older people, but only a small number of subjects in the sample had the condition [148]. Further studies therefore need to be undertaken in large samples of older people with macular degeneration to determine its contribution to falls risk.

Glaucoma

Glaucoma is the name given to the group of eye diseases characterized by an increase in intraocular pressure, which causes pathological changes in the optic disk and associated visual field defects. Glaucoma is a common cause of blindness in older people and affects approximately 3% of people over the age of 65 [146]. The presence of glaucoma has been reported to be associated with an increased risk of falling in both retrospective [26] and prospective investigations [148]. Topical treatments for glaucoma may also increase falls risk. Glynn et al. [151] reported that the use of pupil-constricting eye medications was associated with a threefold increased risk of falling in 489 patients with glaucoma, compared with those patients not using these medications.

Few investigations have been performed to determine the mechanisms underlying eye diseases and falls. It is assumed that the deficits in visual acuity, depth perception and contrast sensitivity and reductions in the size of the visual field associated with these conditions lead to impaired visual judgements of the sur-rounding environment, making the older person more susceptible to tripping over obstacles. Impaired vision has also been associated with slowed gait velocity [152], which is in itself a falls risk factor [153–155]. Furthermore, there is some evidence to suggest that older people rely on visual cues (particularly contrast sensitivity) more than younger people to maintain standing posture [156]. With regard to glaucoma, it has been demonstrated that intraocular pressure increases when transferring from a supine to sitting position, and that this postural change is asso-ciated with further short-term visual impairment [157]. This suggests that older people with glaucoma may be at particular risk of falling when rising from bed.

Lower extremity problems

Osteoarthritis

Osteoarthritis is a common degenerative disease of articular cartilage which pri-marily affects the major weight-bearing joints of the lower limb, leading to struc-tural deformity, decreased range of motion, and pain. A recent epidemiological study in Australia found osteoarthritis to be the commonest cause of muscu-loskeletal disability among older people [158]. Older people with knee and hip osteoarthritis often suffer wasting of associated muscle groups and have difficulty rising from a chair and performing daily tasks, and tend to walk more slowly than older people without the condition [159,160]. There is also evidence to suggest that the presence of osteoarthritis impairs standing balance [161] and joint position sense [162]. It has previously been shown that adequate joint range of motion in the lower limbs is essential to respond adequately to unexpected postural perturba-tions [163, 164], while the presence of pain in lower limb joints may be a source of postural disturbance during voluntary movements. Thus it is clear that osteoarthri-tis, by reducing joint range of motion, reducing muscle strength and causing pain in lower limb joints, will have a detrimental effect on postural stability in older people. A medical history of osteoarthritis has been found to be a significant risk factor for falling by several prospective investigations [1, 3, 4, 26, 34, 165–167], while self-reported symptoms commonly associated with the condition, such as pain or reduced range of motion in the knees and hips, are also associated with increased falls risk [3, 4, 86].

Foot problems

Foot problems are common in older people, affecting at least one in three com-munity-dwelling people over the age of 65 years [168–170], and up to 85% of older people in long-term care facilities [171, 172]. Foot problems may result from osteoarthritic decreases in joint range of motion [173, 174], dermatological conditions [175], detrimental effects of footwear [176–179], and systemic diseases such as peripheral vascular disease [180], diabetes mellitus [181–183] and osteoarthritis [184, 185]. The most commonly reported foot problems in older people are painful corns and calluses, hallux valgus ('bunions'), and hammertoes. Women report a higher prevalence of foot problems than men. The influence of fashion footwear has been found to contribute to foot problems due to the detrimental effect of high heels and a narrow toe-box [176–179, 186].

Foot problems are well recognized as a contributing factor to mobility impairment in older people. Older people with foot pain walk more slowly than those without, and have more difficulty performing daily household tasks [187, 188]. Twenty per cent of older people who are housebound attribute their impaired mobility to foot problems [167], and there is some evidence that assessment of impaired foot and leg function can provide an accurate indicator of overall functional capability, and predict risk of nursing home admission [187].

As the foot provides the structural foundation for both static support and progression of the body during locomotion, it is plausible that foot problems could increase the risk of falling [189, 190]. However, few studies have directly investigated the role of foot problems in postural stability and falls. Two retrospective studies suggested that undefined foot problems were more common in older people who had fallen [86, 191], whereas results from prospective studies have found foot problems (including bunions, hammertoes and ulcers) to only moderately increase risk of falling [26, 52, 164, 192, 193]. One of the limitations with the available evidence is that foot problems are generally poorly defined in epidemiological falls studies, in many cases being coded as a single variable (i.e. presence or absence) or clustered together with other leg problems. This makes it difficult to delineate the contribution of specific foot conditions to falls. Additional research is required to clarify whether specific foot conditions affect balance ability in older people, and whether treatment of foot problems can decrease risk of falling [194].

Urinary incontinence

Incontinence is an extremely common problem in older people, particularly older women. In industrialized societies, up to 34% of older men and 55% of older women suffer from an inability to control urinary functions [195]. Risk factors for incontinence include multiparity, older age, obesity, previous surgery for incontinence, and neurological disorders [196]. Both retrospective and prospective falls investigations have consistently reported urinary incontinence to be a strong risk factor for falls in community-dwelling [4, 34, 192, 197–201] and institutionalized [1, 202, 203] older people.

Falls related to incontinence are generally thought to result from loss of balance when rushing to the toilet or an increased likelihood of slipping on urine. However, there is some question as to whether incontinence is a primary cause of falls, or whether it is simply a marker of generalized physical frailty. While numerous falls in long-term care facilities occur when going to, or returning from the toilet [204], few falls in community-dwelling older people involve toileting. The close associations reported between incontinence, depression, falls and level of mobility suggests that these 'geriatric symptoms' may have shared risk factors rather than causal connections [205].

Psychological and cognitive factors

The role of psychological factors in the predisposition to falls has received comparatively little attention in comparison with common medical problems or sensory and motor function. Perhaps the most widely accepted psychological risk factor for falls is dementia, which affects approximately 6–10% of community-dwelling older people [206] and has been reported as a strong risk factor by numerous investigators [165, 207–212]. Falls related to dementia are of particular concern in long-term care facilities, as cognitive impairment is one of the most common reasons for initial nursing home admission [213]. Furthermore, it has been reported that older people with dementia have a fourfold increased risk of suffering a hip fracture as a result of a fall [165], and a threefold increase in 6-month mortality rate following hip fracture compared with older people without dementia [214].

Cognitive impairment associated with dementia and acute confusional states may increase risk of falling by directly influencing the older person's ability to deal appropriately with environmental hazards, increasing the tendency of an older person to wander [215], and altering gait patterns [216]. In a study of 60 older women with Alzheimer's disease, Brody et al. [217] reported that risk of falling was greatest in those who had previously been vigorous, but had experienced marked decline over recent months. The tendency of dementia sufferers to wander is of particular concern in nursing home residents who are relocated, as it has been shown that fall rates may double when residents are relocated to a new facility [218].

Depression has also been implicated as a falls risk factor. Fifteen per cent of community-dwelling older people show significant depressive symptoms, with 1–2% exhibiting major depressive disorders [219]. In nursing homes, the prevalence of depression can be as high as 25% [220]. Numerous studies have reported an association between depression and falls. Tinetti et al. [192] found depression to be linked to increased risk of falling in community-dwelling older people, as did Nevitt et al. [4], who reported that severe depression was associated with an increased risk of experiencing multiple falls. Subsequent investigations support these early observations, suggesting that the presence of depression is associated with an odds ratio of up to 7.5 for experiencing a fall [24, 94, 199, 221, 222]. Furthermore, the use of antidepressant medications has also been reported to be a risk factor in community-dwelling and institutionalized older people (see Chapter 5).

The mechanisms underlying depressive symptoms and falls risk have not been fully assessed; however, it has been suggested that older people who suffer from depression are less likely to be involved in physical activity, and are therefore at greater risk of falls due to reduced muscle strength, coordination and balance [1]. A recent prospective study of 7414 older women reported that those with depression exhibited significantly poorer self-reported health and functional status than those without, and exhibited a higher risk of hip fracture [222].

Conclusion

In this chapter we have briefly discussed medical conditions most commonly associated with falls in older people. It is evident that although many conditions have been suggested to increase risk of falling in older people, the literature is somewhat equivocal as to the relative importance of each of these conditions. This highlights the benefits of a functional rather than a purely disease-oriented approach to predicting falls. Attributing a degree of falls risk to a specific medical diagnosis has limitations, because the relative severity of the condition may vary considerably between individuals. Furthermore, deficits in sensory and motor function may be evident in many older people with no recorded medical illnesses. As such, the functional approach to falls risk assessment, which involves direct measurement of physical and mental capabilities, would appear to be a useful and complementary approach to assessing risk of falling.

REFERENCES

1 Tinetti ME, Williams TF, Mayewski R. Fall risk index for elderly patients based on number of chronic disabilities. *American Journal of Medicine* 1986;80:429–34.

2 Prudham D, Evans JG. Factors associated with falls in the elderly: a community study. *Age and Ageing* 1981;10:141–6.

3 Campbell AJ, Borrie MJ, Spears GF. Risk factors for falls in a community-based prospective study of people 70 years and older. *Journal of Gerontology* 1989;44:M112–17.

4 Nevitt MC, Cummings SR, Kidd S, Black D. Risk factors for recurrent nonsyncopal falls. A prospective study. *Journal of the American Medical Association* 1989;261:2663–8.

5 Salgado R, Lord SR, Packer J, Ehrlich F. Factors associated with falling in elderly hospital patients. *Gerontology* 1994;40:325–31.

6 O'Loughlin JL, Robitaille Y, Boivin JF, Suissa S. Incidence of and risk factors for falls and injurious falls among the community-dwelling elderly. *American Journal of Epidemiology* 1993;137:342–54.

7 Herndon JG, Helmick CG, Sattin RW, Stevens JA, DeVito C, Wingo PA. Chronic medical conditions and risk of fall injury events at home in older adults. *Journal of the American Geriatrics Society* 1997;45:739–43.

8 Dolinis J, Harrison JE. Factors associated with falling in older Adelaide residents. Australian and New Zealand *Journal of Public Health* 1997;21:462–8.

9 Moseley A, Wales A, Herbert R, Shurr K, Moore S. Observation and analysis of hemiplegic gait: stance phase. *Australian Journal of Physiotherapy* 1993;39:259–67.

10 Tideiksaar R. *Falling in old age: its prevention and treatment.* New York: Springer-Verlag, 1989.

11 Tanner CM. Epidemiology of Parkinson's disease. *Neurology Clinics* 1992;10:317–29.

12 Martin JP. *The basal ganglia and posture.* London: Pitman, 1967.

13 Gregoric M, Lavric A. Statokinesimetric analysis of the postural control in parkinsonism. *Agressologie* 1977;18:45–8.

14 Kitamura J, Nakagawa H, Iinuma K, et al. Visual influence on center of contact pressure in advanced Parkinson's disease. *Archives of Physical Medicine and Rehabilitation* 1993;74:1107–12.

15 Schieppati M, Nardone A. Free and supported stance in Parkinson's disease. *Brain* 1991;114:1227–31.

16 Rogers MW. Disorders of posture, balance, and gait in Parkinson's disease. *Clinics in Geriatric Medicine* 1995;12:825–45.

17 Morris ME, Iansek R, Matyas TA, Summers JJ. The pathogenesis of gait hypokinesia in Parkinson's disease. *Brain* 1994;117:1169–81.

18 Morris ME, Iansek R, Matyas TA, Summers JJ. Stride length regulation in Parkinson's disease. Normalization strategies and underlying mechanisms. *Brain* 1996;119:551–68.

19 Morris M, Iansek R, Matyas T, Summers J. Abnormalities in the stride length-cadence relation in parkinsonian gait. *Movement Disorders* 1998;13:61–9.

20 Smithson F, Morris ME, Iansek R. Performance on clinical tests of balance in Parkinson's disease. *Physical Therapy* 1998;78:577–92.

21 Paulson GW, Schaefer K, Hallum B. Avoiding mental changes and falls in older Parkinson's patients. *Geriatrics* 1986;41:59–62.

22 Koller WC, Glatt S, Vetere-Overfield B, Hassanein R. Falls and Parkinson's disease. *Clinical Neuropharmacology* 1989;12:98–105.

23 Burns R. Falling and getting up again. *Parkinson Report* 1994;XV:18.

24 Granek E, Baker SP, Abbey H, et al. Medications and diagnoses in relation to falls in a long-term care facility. *Journal of the American Geriatrics Society* 1987;35:503–11.

25 Studenski S, Duncan PW, Chandler J, et al. Predicting falls: the role of mobility and non-physical factors. *Journal of the American Geriatrics Society* 1994;42:297–302.

26 Dolinis J, Harrison JE, Andrews GR. Factors associated with falling in older Adelaide residents. *Australian and New Zealand Journal of Public Health* 1997;21:462–8.

27 Brain R, Northfield D, Wilkinson M. Neurological manifestations of cervical spondylosis. *Brain* 1952;75:187–225.

28 Sudarsky L, Ronthal M. Gait disorders among elderly patients. A survey study of 50 patients. *Archives of Neurology* 1983;40:740–3.

29 Dichgans J, Mauritz KH, Allum JHJ, Brandt T. Postural sway in normals and ataxic patients. *Aggressologie* 1976;17C:15–24.

30 Mauritz KH, Dichgans J, Hufschmidt A. Quantitative analysis of stance in late cortical cerebellar atrophy of the anterior lobe and other forms of cerebellar ataxia. *Brain* 1979;102:461–82.

31 Bronstein AM, Hood JD, Gresty MA, Panagi C. Visual control of balance in cerebellar and parkinsonian syndromes. *Brain* 1990;113:767–79.

32 Horak FB, Diener HC. Cerebellar control of postural scaling and central set in stance. *Journal of Neurophysiology* 1994;72:479–93.

33 Diener HC, Nutt JG. Vestibular and cerebellar disorders of equilibrium and gait. In: Masdeu JC, Sudarsky L, Wolfson L, editors. *Gait disorders of aging: falls and therapeutic strategies.* Philadelphia: Lippincott-Raven, 1997:261–72.

34 Robbins AS, Rubenstein LZ, Josephson KR, Schulman BL, Osterweil D, Fine G. Predictors of falls among elderly people – results of two population-based studies. *Archives of Internal Medicine* 1989;149:1628–33.

35 Gehlsen GM, Whaley MH. Falls in the elderly, Part I. Gait. *Archives of Physical Medicine and Rehabilitation* 1990;71:735–8.

36 Woolley SM, Czaja SJ, Drury CG. An assessment of falls in elderly men and women. *Journal of Gerontology* 1997;52A:M80–7.

37 Lord SR, Lloyd DG, Li SK. Sensori-motor function, gait patterns and falls in community-dwelling women. *Age and Ageing* 1996;25:292–9.

38 Hausdorff JM, Edelberg HK, Mitchell SL, Goldberger AL, Wei JY. Increased gait unsteadiness in community-dwelling elderly fallers. *Archives of Physical Medicine and Rehabilitation* 1997;78:278–83.

39 Maki BE. Gait changes in older adults: predictors of falls or indicators of fear? *Journal of the American Geriatrics Society* 1997;45:313–20.

40 Kroenke K, Lucas CA, Rosenberg ML, et al. Causes of persistent dizziness. A prospective study of 100 patients in ambulatory care. Annals of Internal Medicine 1992;117:898–904.

41 Fife TD, Baloh RW: Disequilibrium of unknown cause in older people. *Annals of Neurology* 1993;34:694–702.

42 Lord SR, Clark RD, Webster IW. Physiological factors associated with falls in an elderly population. *Journal of the American Geriatrics Society* 1991;39:1194–200.

43 Lord SR, Ward JA, Williams P, Anstey KJ. Physiological factors associated with falls in older community-dwelling women. *Journal of the American Geriatrics Society* 1994;42:1110–17.

44 Lord SR, Webster IW. Visual field dependence in elderly fallers and non-fallers. *International Journal of Aging and Human Development* 1990;31:267–77.

45 Brandt T, Dieterich M. Vestibular falls. *Journal of Vestibular Research* 1993;3:3–14.

46 Lawson J, Fitzgerald J, Birchall J, Aldren CP, Kenny RA. Diagnosis of geriatric patients with severe dizziness. *Journal of the American Geriatrics Society* 1999;47:7–12.

47 Lipsitz LA, Jonsson PV, Kelley MM, Koestner JS. Causes and correlates of recurrent falls in ambulatory frail elderly. *Journal of Gerontology* 1991;46:M114–22.

48 Sorock GS, Labiner DM. Peripheral neuromuscular dysfunction and falls in an elderly cohort. *American Journal of Epidemiology* 1992;136:584–91.

49 Hurley MV, Rees J, Newham DJ. Quadriceps function, proprioceptive acuity and functional performance in healthy young, middle-aged and elderly subjects. *Age and Ageing* 1998;27:55–62.

50 Era P, Heikkinen E. Postural sway during standing and unexpected disturbance of balance in random samples of men of different ages. *Journal of Gerontology* 1985;40:287–95.

51 Era P, Schroll M, Ytting H, Gause-Nilsson I, Heikkinen E, Steen B. Postural balance and its sensory-motor correlates in 75-year-old men and women: a cross-national comparative study. *Journal of Gerontology* 1996;51:M53–63.

52 Koski K, Luukinen H, Laippala P, Kivela S-L. Risk factors for major injurious falls among the home-dwelling elderly by functional abilities. *Gerontology* 1998;44:232–8.

53 Sabin TD. Peripheral neuropathy: disorders of proprioception. In: Masdeu JC, Sudarsky L, Wolfson L, editors. *Gait disorders of aging: falls and therapeutic strategies.* Philadelphia: Lippincott – Raven, 1997:273–82.

54 Pirart J. Diabetes mellitus and its degenerative complications: a prospective study of 4440 patients observed between 1947 and 1973. *Diabetes Care* 1979;2:168–88.

55 Simoneau GG, Ulbrecht JS, Derr JA, Becker MB, Cavanagh PR. Postural instability in patients with diabetic sensory neuropathy. *Diabetes Care* 1994;17:1411–21.

56 Uccioli L, Giacomini P, Magrini A, et al. Body sway in diabetic neuropathy. *Diabetes Care* 1995;18:339–44.

57 Richardson JK, Ashton-Miller JA, Lee SG, Jacobs K. Moderate peripheral neuropathy impairs weight transfer and unipedal balance in the elderly. *Archives of Physical Medicine and Rehabilitation* 1996;77:1152–6.

58 VandenBosch C, Gilsing M, Lee S-G, Richardson J, Ashton-Miller J. Peripheral neuropathy effect on ankle inversion and eversion detection thresholds. *Archives of Physical Medicine and Rehabilitation* 1995;76:850–6.

59 Simoneau GG, Derr JA, Ulbrecht JS, Becker MB, Cavanagh PR. Diabetic sensory neuropathy effect on ankle joint movement perception. *Archives of Physical Medicine and Rehabilitation* 1996;77:453–60.

60 Cavanagh P, Derr J, Ulbrecht J, Maser R, Orchard T. Problems with gait and posture in neuropathic patients with insulin-dependent diabetes mellitus. *Diabetic Medicine* 1992;9:469–74.

61 Richardson JK, Ching C, Hurvitz EA. The relationship between electromyographically documented peripheral neuropathy and falls. *Journal of the American Geriatrics Society* 1992;40:1008–12.

62 Richardson JK, Hurvitz EA. Peripheral neuropathy: a true risk factor for falls. *Journal of Gerontology* 1995;50:M211–15.

63 Rutan GH, Hermanson B, Bild DE, Kittner SL, LaBaw F, Tell GS. Orthostatic hypotension

in older adults: the cardiovascular health study. *Journal of the American Geriatrics Society* 1992;40:1079–80.

64 Kwok T, Liddle J, Hastie IR. Postural hypotension and falls. *Postgraduate Medical Journal* 1995;71:278–80.

65 Rodstein M, Zeman F. Postural blood pressure changes in the elderly. *Journal of Chronic Diseases* 1957;6:581–8.

66 Johnson RH, Smith AC, Spalding JMK. Effect of posture on blood pressure in elderly patients. *Lancet* 1965;I:731–3.

67 Caird FI, Andrews GR, Kennedy RD. Effect of posture on blood pressure in the elderly. *British Heart Journal* 1973;35:527–30.

68 Myers MG, Kearns PM, Kennedy DS, Fisher RH. Postural hypotension and diuretic therapy in the elderly. *Canadian Medical Association Journal* 1978;119:581–4.

69 Lennox IM, Williams BO. Postural hypotension in the elderly. *Clinical and Experimental Gerontology* 1980;2:313–29.

70 Palmer KT. Studies into postural hypotension in elderly patients. *New Zealand Medical Journal* 1983;96:43–5.

71 Aronow WS, Lee NH, Sales FF, Etienne F. Prevalence of postural hypotension in elderly patients in a long-term health care facility. *American Journal of Cardiology* 1988;62:336.

72 Burke V, Beilin LJ, German R, et al. Postural fall in blood pressure in the elderly in relation to drug treatment and other lifestyle factors. *Quarterly Journal of Medicine* 1992;84:583–91.

73 Raiha I, Luutonen S, Piha J, Seppanen A, Toikka T, Sourander L. Prevalence, predisposing factors, and prognostic importance of postural hypotension. *Archives of Internal Medicine* 1995;155:930–5.

74 Tilvis RS, Hakala SM, Valvanne J, Erkinjuntti T. Postural hypotension and dizziness in a general aged population: a four-year follow-up of the Helsinki Aging Study. *Journal of the American Geriatrics Society* 1996;44:809–14.

75 Masaki KH, Schatz IJ, Burchfiel CM, et al. Orthostatic hypotension predicts mortality in elderly men: the Honolulu Heart Program. *Circulation* 1998;98:2290–5.

76 Mader SL, Josephson KR, Rubenstein LZ. Low prevalence of postural hypotension among community-dwelling elderly. *Journal of the American Medical Association* 1987;258:1511–14.

77 Low PA, Opfer-Gehrking TL, McPhee BR, et al. Prospective evaluation of clinical characteristics of orthostatic hypotension. *Mayo Clinic Proceedings* 1995;70:617–22.

78 Mathias CJ. Orthostatic hypotension: causes, mechanisms, and influencing factors. *Neurology* 1995;45:S6–11.

79 Tivlis RS, Hakala SM, Valvanne J, Erkinjuntti T. Postural hypotension and dizziness in a general aged population: a four year follow-up of the Helsinki aging study. *Journal of the American Geriatrics Society* 1996;44:809–14.

80 Hillen ME, Wagner ML, Sage JI. 'Subclinical' orthostatic hypotension is associated with dizziness in elderly patients with Parkinson's disease. *Archives of Physical Medicine and Rehabilitation* 1996;77:710–12.

81 Mets TF. Drug-induced orthostatic hypotension in older patients. *Drugs and Aging* 1995;6:219–28.

82 Luutonen S, Neuvonen P, Ruskoaho H, et al. The role of potassium in postural hypotension:

electrolytes and neurohumoral factors in elderly hypertensive patients using diuretics. *Journal of Internal Medicine* 1995;237:375–80.

83 Dambrink JH, Wieling W. Circulatory response to postural change in healthy male subjects in relation to age. *Clinical Science* 1987;72:335–41.

84 Sheldon JH. On the natural history of falls in old age. *British Medical Journal* 1960;ii1685–1690.

85 Campbell AJ, Reinken J, Allan BC, Martinez GS. Falls in old age: a study of frequency and related clinical factors. *Age and Ageing* 1981;10:264–70.

86 Gabell A, Simons MA, Nayak USL. Falls in the healthy elderly: predisposing causes. *Ergonomics* 1985;28:965–75.

87 Rubenstein LZ, Robbins AS, Josephson KR, Schulman BL, Osterweil D. The value of assessing falls in an elderly population. A randomized clinical trial. *Annals of Internal Medicine* 1990;113:308–16.

88 Jonsson PV, Lipsitz LA, Kelley M, Koestner J. Hypotensive responses to common daily activities in institutionalized elderly. A potential risk for recurrent falls. *Archives of Internal Medicine* 1990;150:1518–24.

89 Brocklehurst JC, Exton-Smith AN, Lempert Barber SM, Hunt LP, Palmer MK. Fracture of the femur in old age: A two-centre study of associated clinical factors and the cause of the fall. *Age and Ageing* 1978;7:2–15.

90 Kirshen AJ, Cape RDT, Hayes HC, Spencer JD. Postural sway and cardiovascular parameters associated with falls in the elderly. *Journal of Clinical Experimental Gerontology* 1984;6:291–307.

91 Lord SR, Clark RD, Webster IW. Physiological factors associated with falls in an elderly population. In: Beck, JC, et al., editors *Year book of geriatrics and gerontology* 1993. St Louis: Mosby, 1993.

92 Lord SR, Anstey KJ, Williams P, Ward JA. Psychoactive medication use, sensori-motor function and falls in older women. *British Journal of Clinical Pharmacology* 1995;39:227–34.

93 Clark RD, Lord SR, Webster IW. Clinical parameters associated with falls in an elderly population. *Gerontology* 1993;39:117–23.

94 Liu BA, Topper AK, Reeves RA, Gryfe C, Maki BE: Falls among older people: relationship to medication use and orthostatic hypotension. *Journal of the American Geriatrics Society* 1995;43:1141–5.

95 Consensus statement on the definition of orthostatic hypotension, pure autonomic failure, and multiple system atrophy. *Journal of Neurological Sciences* 1996;144:218–19.

96 Rutan GH, Hermanson B, Bild DE, Kittner SJ, LaBaw F, Tell GS. Orthostatic hypotension in older adults. The cardiovascular health study: CHS Collaborative Research Group. *Hypertension* 1992;19:508–19.

97 Lipsitz LA, Storch HA, Minaker KL, Rowe JW. Intra-individual variability in postural blood pressure in the elderly. *Clinical Science* 1985;69:337–41.

98 Ward C, Kenny RA. Reproducibility of orthostatic hypotension in symptomatic elderly. *American Journal of Medicine* 1996;100:418–22.

99 Lipsitz LA. Abnormalities in blood pressure homeostasis that contribute to falls in the elderly. *Clinics in Geriatric Medicine* 1985;1:637–48.

100 Jansen RWMM, Connelly CM, Kelley-Gagnon MM, Parker JA, Lipsitz LA. Postprandial hypotension in elderly patients with unexplained syncope. *Archives of Internal Medicine* 1995;155:945–52.

101 Peitzman SJ, Berger SR. Postprandial blood pressure decrease in well elderly persons. *Archives of Internal Medicine* 1989;149:286–8.

102 Aronow WS, Ahn C. Postprandial hypotension in 499 elderly persons in a long-term health care facility. *Journal of the American Geriatrics Society* 1994;42:930–2.

103 Blumenthal MD, Davie JW. Dizziness and falling in elderly psychiatric outpatients. *American Journal of Psychiatry* 1980;137:203–6.

104 Ensrud KE, Nevitt MC, Yunis C, Hulley SB, Grimm RH, Cummings SR. Postural hypotension and postural dizziness in elderly women. The study of osteoporotic fractures. The Study of Osteoporotic Fractures Research Group. *Archives of Internal Medicine* 1992;152:1058–64.

105 Craig GM. Clinical presentation of orthostatic hypotension in the elderly. *Postgraduate Medical Journal* 1994;70:638–42.

106 Sloane PD, Dallara J. Clinical research and geriatric dizziness: the blind men and the elephant. *Journal of the American Geriatrics Society* 1999;47:113–14.

107 Lipsitz LA. The drop attack: a common geriatric symptom. *Journal of the American Geriatrics Society* 1983;31:617–20.

108 Meissner I, Wiebers DO, Swanson JW, O'Fallon WM. The natural history of drop attacks. *Neurology* 1986;36:1029–34.

109 Sheehan S, Bauer RB, Meyer JS. Vertebral artery compression in cervical spondylosis: arteriographic demonstration during life of vertebral artery insufficiency due to rotation and extension of the neck. *Neurology* 1960;10:968–72.

110 Williams D, Wilson TG. The diagnosis of major and minor syndromes of basilar insufficiency. *Brain* 1962;85:741–7.

111 Kubala MJ, Millikan CH. Diagnosis, pathogenesis, and treatment of 'drop attacks'. *Archives of Neurology* 1964;11:107–10.

112 Kameyama M. Vertigo and drop attack. With special reference to cerebrovascular disorders and atherosclerosis of the vertebral–basilar system. *Geriatrics* 1965;20:892–900.

113 Brust JCM, Plank CR, Healton EB. The pathology of drop attacks: a case report. *Neurology* 1979;29:786–8.

114 Kremer M. Sitting, standing and walking. *British Medical Journal* 1958;ii:121.

115 VanNorel GJ, Verhagen WI. Drop attacks and instability of the degenerate cervical spine. *Journal of Bone and Joint Surgery (Br)* 1996;78:495–6.

116 Walter PF, Crawley IS, Dorney ER. Carotid sinus hypersensitivity and syncope. *Neurology* 1978;27:746–51.

117 Murphy AL, Rowbotham BJ, Boyle RS, Thew CM, Fardoulys JA, Wilson K. Carotid sinus hypersensitivity in elderly nursing home patients. *Australian and New Zealand Journal of Medicine* 1986;16:24–7.

118 Kenny RA, Traynor G. Carotid sinus syndrome: clinical characteristics in elderly patients. *Age and Ageing* 1991;20:449–54.

119 Dey AB, Stout NR, Kenny RA. Cardiovascular syncope is the most common cause of drop attacks in the elderly. *Pacing and Clinical Electrophysiology* 1997;20:818–19.

120 Odkvist LM, Bergenius J. Drop attacks in Menière's disease. *Acta Otolaryngologica Supplementum* 1988;455:82–5.

121 Baloh RW, Jacobson K, Winder T. Drop attacks with Menière's syndrome. *Annals of Neurology* 1990;28:384–7.

122 Fukushima K, Fujiwara T, Yagi K, Seino M. Drop attacks and epileptic syndromes. *Japanese Journal of Psychiatry and Neurology* 1993;47:211–16.

123 Tinuper P, Cerullo A, Marini C, et al. Epileptic drop attacks in partial epilepsy: clinical features, evolution, and prognosis. *Journal of Neurology, Neurosurgery and Psychiatry* 1998;64:231–7.

124 Clark AN. Factors in fracture of the female femur. A clinical study of the environmental, physical, medical and preventive aspects of this injury. *Gerontologica Clinica* 1968;10:257–70.

125 Stevens DL, Matthews WB. Cryptogenic drop attacks: an affliction of women. *British Medical Journal* 1973;i:439–42.

126 Overstall PW, Exton-Smith AN, Imms FJ, Johnson AL. Falls in the elderly related to postural imbalance. *British Medical Journal* 1977;i:261–4.

127 Davies AJ, Kenny RA. Falls presenting to the accident and emergency department: types of presentation and risk factor profile. *Age and Ageing* 1996;25:362–6.

128 Richardson DA, Bexton RS, Shaw FE, Kenny RA. Prevalence of cardioinhibitory carotid sinus hypersensitivity in patients 50 years or over presenting to the accident and emergency department with 'unexplained' or 'recurrent' falls. *Pacing and Clinical Electrophysiology* 1997;20:820–3.

129 Smiddy J, Lewis HD, Dunn M. The effect of carotid massage in older men. *Journal of Gerontology* 1972;27:209–11.

130 Lipsitz LA. Syncope in the elderly. *Annals of Internal Medicine* 1983;99:92–105.

131 Kapoor W, Snustad D, Peterson J, Wieand H, Cha R, Karpf M. Syncope in the elderly. *American Journal of Medicine* 1986;80:419–28.

132 Jansen RWMM, Lenders JWM, Thien T, Hoefnagels WHI. Antihypertensive treatment and post-prandial blood pressure reduction in the elderly. *Gerontology* 1987;95:363–8.

133 Micieli G, Martignoni E, Cavallini A, Sandrini G, Nappi G. Postprandial and orthostatic hypotension in Parkinson's disease. *Neurology* 1987;37:386–93.

134 Robertson D, Wade D, Robertson RM. Postprandial alterations in cardiovascular hemodynamics in autonomic dysfunctional states. *American Journal of Cardiology* 1981;48:1048–52.

135 O'Mahony D, Foote C. Prospective evaluation of unexplained syncope, dizziness, and falls among community-dwelling elderly adults. *Journal of Gerontology* 1998;53:M435–40.

136 Lawson J, Fitzgerald J, Birchall J, Aldren CP, Kenny RA. Diagnosis of geriatric patients with severe dizziness. *Journal of the American Geriatrics Society* 1999;47:12–17.

137 Shaw FE, Kenny RA. The overlap between syncope and falls in the elderly. *Postgraduate Medical Journal* 1997;73:635–9.

138 Nevitt MC, Cummings SR, Hudes ES. Risk factors for injurious falls: a prospective study. *Journal of Gerontology* 1991;46:M164–70.

139 Sekuler R, Kline D, Dismukes K, editors. *Aging and human visual function.* New York: Liss, 1982.

140 Gittings NS, Fozard JL. Age related changes in visual acuity. *Experimental Gerontology* 1986;21:423–33.

141 Lord SR, Clark RD, Webster IW. Visual acuity and contrast sensitivity in relation to falls in an elderly population. *Age and Ageing* 1991;2:175–81.

142 Lord SR, McLean D, Stathers G. Physiological factors associated with injurious falls in older people living in the community. *Gerontology* 1992;38:338–46.

143 Jack CI, Smith T, Neoh C, Lye M, McGalliard JN. Prevalence of low vision in elderly patients admitted to an acute geriatric unit in Liverpool: elderly people who fall are more likely to have low vision. *Gerontology* 1995;41:280–5.

144 Lord SR, Ward JA, Williams P, Anstey KJ. An epidemiological study of falls in older community-dwelling women: the Randwick falls and fractures study. *Australian Journal of Public Health* 1993;17:240–5.

145 Spector A. Aging of the lens and cataract formation. In: Sekular R, Kline D, Dismukes K, editors. *Aging and human visual function.* New York: Liss, 1982;27–43.

146 Kahn HA, Leibowitz HM, Ganley JP, et al. The Framingham eye study. I. Outline and major prevalence findings. *American Journal of Epidemiology* 1977;106:17–32.

147 Felson DT, Anderson JJ, Hannan MT, Milton RC, Wilson PW, Kiel DP. Impaired vision and hip fracture. The Framingham study. *Journal of the American Geriatrics Society* 1989;37: 495–500.

148 Ivers RQ, Cumming RG, Mitchell P, Attebo K. Visual impairment and falls in older adults: the Blue Mountains eye study. *Journal of the American Geriatrics Society* 1998;46:58–64.

149 Mitchell P, Smith W, Attebo K, Wang JJ. Prevalence of age-related maculopathy in Australia: the Blue Mountains eye study. *Ophthalmology* 1995;102:1450–60.

150 Vingerling JR, Klaver CCW, Hoffman A, DeJong TVM. Epidemiology of age-related maculopathy. *Epidemiological Reviews* 1995;17:347–60.

151 Glynn RJ, Seddon JM, Krug JH, Jr, Sahagian CR, Chiavelli ME, Campion EW. Falls in elderly patients with glaucoma. *Archives of Ophthalmology* 1991;109:205–10.

152 Klein BE, Klein R, Lee KE, Cruickshanks KJ. Performance-based and self-assessed measures of visual function as related to history of falls, hip fractures, and measured gait time. The Beaver Dam eye study. *Ophthalmology* 1998;105:160–4.

153 Guimaraes RM, Isaacs B. Characteristics of the gait in old people who fall. *International Rehabilitation Medicine* 1980;2:177–80.

154 Wolfson L, Whipple R, Amerman P, Tobin JN. Gait assessment in the elderly: a gait abnormality rating scale and its relation to falls. *Journal of Gerontology* 1990;45:M12–19.

155 Cho CY, Kamen G. Detecting balance deficits in frequent fallers using clinical and quantitative evaluation tools. *Journal of the American Geriatrics Society* 1998;46:426–30.

156 Turano K, Rubin GS, Herdman SJ, Chee E, Fried LP. Visual stabilization of posture in the elderly: fallers versus nonfallers. *Optometry and Vision Science* 1994;71:761–9.

157 Lietz A, Kaiser HJ, Stumpfig D, Flammer J. Influence of posture on the visual field in glaucoma patients and controls. *Ophthalmologica* 1995;209:129–31.

158 March LM, Brnabic AJ, Skinner JC, Schwarz JM. Musculoskeletal disability among elderly people in the community. *Medical Journal of Australia* 1998;168:439–42.

159 Gibbs J, Hughes S, Dunlop D, Singer R, Chang R. Predictors of change in walking velocity in older adults. *Journal of the American Geriatrics Society* 1996;44:126–32.

160 Hurley MV, Scott DL, Rees J, Newham DJ. Sensorimotor changes and functional performance in patients with knee osteoarthritis. *Annals of the Rheumatic Diseases* 1997;56:641–8.

161 Wegener L, Kisner C, Nichols D. Static and dynamic balance responses in persons with bilateral knee osteoarthritis. *Journal of Orthopaedic and Sports Physical Therapy* 1997;25:13–18.

162 Pai YC, Rymer WZ, Chang RW, Sharma L. Effect of age and osteoarthritis on knee proprioception. *Arthritis and Rheumatism* 1997;40:2260–5.

163 Studenski S, Duncan PW, Chandler J. Postural responses and effector factors in persons with unexplained falls: results and methodologic issues. *Journal of the American Geriatrics Society* 1991;39:229–34.

164 Whipple R, Wolfson L, Derby C, Singh D, Tobin J. Altered sensory function and balance in older persons. *Journal of Gerontology* 1993;48:71–6.

166 Blake A, Morgan K, Bendall M, et al. Falls by elderly people at home – prevalence and associated factors. *Age and Ageing* 1988;17:365–72.

167 Buchner DM, Larson EB. Falls and fractures in patients with Alzheimer-type dementia. *Journal of the American Medical Association* 1987;257:1492–5.

168 Black JR, Hale WE. Prevalence of foot complaints in the elderly. *Journal of the American Podiatric Medical Association* 1987;77:308–11.

169 White E, Mulley G. Footcare for very elderly people: a community survey. *Age and Ageing* 1989;18:275–8.

170 Harvey I, Frankel S, Marks R, Shalom D, Morgan M. Foot morbidity and exposure to chiropody: population based study. *British Medical Journal* 1997;315:1054–5.

171 Hung L, Ho Y, Leung P. Survey of foot deformities among 166 geriatric inpatients. *Foot and Ankle* 1985;5:156–64.

172 Helfand AE, Cooke HL, Walinsky MD, Demp PH. Foot problems associated with older patients: a focused podogeriatric study. *Journal of the American Podiatric Medical Association* 1998;88:237–41.

173 Nigg B, Fisher V, Allinger T, Ronsky J, Engsberg J. Range of motion of the foot as a function of age. *Foot and Ankle* 1992;13:336–43.

174 Vandervoort AA, Chesworth BM, Cunningham DA, Paterson DH, Rechnitzer PA, Koval JJ. Age and sex effects on mobility of the human ankle. *Journal of Gerontology* 1992;47:M17–21.

175 Schiralid F. Common dermatologic manifestations in the older patient. *Clinics in Podiatric Medicine and Surgery* 1993;10:79–95.

176 Gorecki G. Shoe-related foot problems and public health. *Journal of the American Podiatry Association* 1978;4:245–7.

177 Chung S. Foot care – a health care maintenance programme. *Journal of Gerontological Nursing* 1983;9:213–27.

178 Herman H, Bottomly J. Anatomical and biomechanical considerations of the elder foot. *Topics in Geriatric Rehabilitation* 1992;7:1–13.

179 Frey C, Thompson F, Smith J, Sanders M, Horstman H. American Orthopaedic Foot and Ankle Society women's shoe survey. *Foot and Ankle* 1993;14:78–81.

180 Robbins J, Austin C. Common peripheral vascular diseases. *Clinics in Podiatric Medicine and Surgery* 1993;10:205–19.

181 Green D. Acute and chronic complications of diabetes mellitus in older patients. *American Journal of Medicine* 1986;80:39–45.

182 Jacobs A. Diabetes mellitus. *Clinics in Podiatric Medicine and Surgery* 1993;10:231–48.

183 Benbow SJ, Walsh A, Gill GV. Diabetes in institutionalised elderly people: a forgotten population? *British Medical Journal* 1997;314:1868.

184 D'Amico J. The pathomechanics of adult rheumatoid arthritis affecting the foot. *Journal of the American Podiatry Association* 1976;66:227–30.

185 Black JR, Cahalin C, Germaine BF. Pedal morbidity in rheumatic disease. *Journal of the American Podiatry Association* 1982;72:360–4.

186 Coughlin MJ. Mallet toes, hammer toes, claw toes and corns. *Postgraduate Medicine* 1984;75:191–8.

187 Guralnik J, Simonsick E, Ferrucci L, et al. A short physical performance battery assessing lower extremity function: association with self-reported disability and prediction of mortality and nursing home admission. *Journal of Gerontology* 1994;49:M85–94.

188 Benvenutti F, Ferrucci L, Guralnik J, Gangemi S, Baroni A. Foot pain and disability in older persons: an epidemiologic survey. *Journal of the American Geriatrics Society* 1995;43:479–84.

189 DeLargy D. Accidents in old people. *Medical Press* 1958;239:117–120.

190 Helfand AE. Foot impairment: an etiologic factor in falls in the aged. *Journal of the American Podiatry Association* 1966;56:326–9.

191 Wild D, Nayak U, Isaacs B. Characteristics of old people who fell at home. *Journal of Clinical and Experimental Gerontology* 1980;2:271–87.

192 Tinetti ME, Speechley M, Ginter SF. Risk factors for falls among elderly persons living in the community. *New England Journal of Medicine* 1988;319:1701–7.

193 Koski K, Luukinen H, Laippala P, Kivela SL. Physiological factors and medications as predictors of injurious falls by elderly people: a prospective population-based study. *Age and Ageing* 1996;25:29–38.

194 Menz HB, Lord SR. Foot problems, functional impairment and falls in older people. *Journal of the American Podiatric Medical Association* 1999;89:458–67.

195 Thom D. Variation in estimates of urinary incontinence prevalence in the community: effects of differences in definition, population characteristics, and study type. *Journal of the American Geriatrics Society* 1998;46:473–80.

196 Gardner J, Fonda D. Urinary incontinence in the elderly. *Disability and Rehabilitation* 1994;16:140–8.

197 Teno J, Kiel DP, Mor V. Multiple stumbles: a risk factor for falls in community-dwelling elderly. A prospective study. *Journal of the American Geriatrics Society* 1990;38:1321–5.

198 Yasumura S, Haga H, Nagai H, Suzuki T, Amano H, Shibata H. Rate of falls and the correlates among elderly people living in an urban community in Japan. *Age and Ageing* 1994;23:323–7.

199 Kutner NG, Schechtman KB, Ory MG, Baker DI. Older adults' perceptions of their health

and functioning in relation to sleep disturbance, falling, and urinary incontinence. *Journal of the American Geriatrics Society* 1994;42:757–62.

200 Luukinen H, Koski K, Kivela SL, Laippala P. Social status, life changes, housing conditions, health, functional abilities and life-style as risk factors for recurrent falls among the home-dwelling elderly. *Public Health* 1996;110:115–18.

201 Tromp AM, Smit JH, Deeg DJ, Bouter LM, Lips P. Predictors of falls and fractures in the longitudinal aging study, Amsterdam. *Journal of Bone and Mineral Research* 1998;12:1932–9.

202 Gluck T, Wientjes HJ, Rai GS. An evaluation of risk factors for inpatient falls in acute and rehabilitation elderly care wards. *Gerontology* 1996;42:104–7.

203 Stevenson B, Mills EM, Welin L, Beal KG. Falls risk factors in an acute-care setting: a retrospective study. *Canadian Journal of Nursing Research* 1998;30:97–111.

204 Ashley MJ, Gryfe CI, Amies A. A longitudinal study of falls in an elderly population II. Some circumstances of falling. *Age and Ageing* 1977;6:211–20.

205 Tinetti ME, Inouye SK, Gill TM, Doucette JT. Shared risk factors for falls, incontinence, and functional dependence. Unifying the approach to geriatric syndromes. *Journal of the American Medical Association* 1995;273:1348–53.

206 Hendrie HC. Epidemiology of dementia and Alzheimer's disease. *American Journal of Geriatric Psychiatry* 1998;62:S3–18.

207 Morris JC, Rubin EH, Morris EJ, Mandel SA. Senile dementia of the Alzheimer's type: an important risk factor for serious falls. *Journal of Gerontology* 1987;42:412–17.

208 Buchner DM, Larson EB. Transfer bias and the association of cognitive impairment with falls. *Journal of General Internal Medicine* 1988;3:254–9.

209 Gross YT, Shimamoto Y, Rose CL, Frank B. Why do they fall? Monitoring risk factors in nursing homes. *Journal of Gerontological Nursing* 1990;16:20–5.

210 Jantti PO, Pyykko VI, Hervonen AL. Falls among elderly nursing home residents. *Public Health* 1993;107:89–96.

211 Asada T, Kariya T, Kinoshita T, et al. Predictors of fall-related injuries among community-dwelling elderly people with dementia. *Age and Ageing* 1996;25:22–8.

212 Johansson C, Skoog I. A population-based study on the association between dementia and hip fractures in 85-year olds. *Aging* 1996;8:189–96.

213 Lord SR. Predictors of nursing home placement and mortality of residents in intermediate care. *Age and Ageing* 1994;23:499–504.

214 Baker BR, Duckworth T, Wilkes E. Mental state and other prognostic factors in femoral fractures of the elderly. *Journal of the Royal College of General Practitioners* 1978;28:557–9.

215 Mossey JM. Social and psychologic factors related to falls among the elderly. *Clinics in Geriatric Medicine* 1985;1:541–53.

216 Nakamura T, Meguro K, Sasaki H. Relationship between falls and stride length variability in senile dementia of the Alzheimer type. *Gerontology* 1996;42:108–13.

217 Brody EM, Kleban MH, Moss MS, Kleban F. Predictors of falls among institutionalized women with Alzheimer's disease. *Journal of the American Geriatrics Society* 1984;32:877–82.

218 Friedman SM, Williamson JD, Lee BH, Ankrom MA, Ryan SD, Denman SJ. Increased fall rates in nursing home residents after relocation to a new facility. *Journal of the American Geriatrics Society* 1995;43:1237–42.

219 Blazer D, Hughes DC. The epidemiology of depression in an elderly community population. *Gerontologist* 1987;27:281–7.

220 Samuels SC, Katz IB. Depression in the nursing home. *Psychiatry Annual* 1995;25:419–24.

221 Myers AH, Baker SP, Van Natta ML, Abbey H, Robinson EG. Risk factors associated with falls and injuries among elderly institutionalized persons. *American Journal of Epidemiology* 1991;133:1179–90.

222 Whooley MA, Kip KE, Cauley JA, Ensrud KE, Nevitt MC, Browner WS. Depression, falls, and risk of fracture in older women. *Archives of Internal Medicine* 1999;158:484–90.

5

Medications as risk factors for falls

By Beth Matters, Hylton B. Menz, Catherine Sherrington and Stephen R. Lord

In the USA and Europe it has been estimated that the aged population account for 25–50% of expenditure on medications [1] with 85% of older people taking at least one medication, and 48% taking three or more [2]. Older people are particularly responsive to the effects of pharmacological treatment, which makes them especially vulnerable to the adverse reactions of many medications [3–5]. It has been well documented that the greater the number of medications taken, the greater the risk of falling [2, 6–16]. Cumming et al. [2] reported that the relative risk of experiencing a fall when using one medication is 1.4, two medications 2.2, and three or more medications 2.4. Although multiple drug use may be partly a proxy measure for poor health, there is increasing evidence that multiple medication use may lead to falls as a result of adverse reactions to one or more medication, detrimental drug interactions, and/or incorrect use [17].

While the relationship between polypharmacy and falls is well established, the relationship between specific classes of drugs and risk of falling is not as clear. The following drug groups have most commonly been implicated in the aetiology of falls: psychoactive medications (including hypnotics and anxiolytics, antidepressants and antipsychotics), cardiovascular medications (including antihypertensives, diuretics and vasodilators), analgesics and anti-inflammatories [4]. However, before reviewing the studies that have looked for possible causal relationships between each of the above medication classes and falls, it is worth examining the study design issues and other limiting factors which make this area of study notoriously difficult.

Design issues and limiting factors

Limitations observed in most current study designs include confounding by indication, small sample sizes and questionable reliability and validity. Confounding by indication makes it impossible to ascertain whether the relationship between falls and medication is due to the actual drugs, or the indications for their use. Such confounders include disease, depression, anxiety and impaired cognitive status.

While early studies failed to address possible confounding factors, more recent studies have taken this into account [2]. Due to small sample sizes, many studies have been unable to explore the effects of individual medications grouped within drug classes [11, 17, 18]. Retrospective studies have come under criticism for their lack of reliability and validity. Many involve the subjective recall of a falls event, which is questionable as up to one-third of older people forget about experiencing a fall 3 months to 1 year later [19]. Furthermore, drug use may change over time, and a fall may lead to a change in the older person's medication [17, 20].

Despite these considerable impediments, many studies have now been undertaken in this area and patterns of evidence are emerging which indicate that some drug classes are indeed implicated in increasing falls risk in older people, whereas others are not. The following sections review this material.

Drug classes implicated in falls in older people

Psychoactive medications

Many epidemiological studies have examined the association between the use of any psychoactive medication and falls and falls injuries in older people. These studies indicate that there is a two- to threefold increased risk of falling when using psychoactive medications [9, 21–26], and a twofold increased risk of experiencing a hip fracture [27]. The use of multiple psychoactive medications also has an additive effect on falls risk. For example, Weiner et al. [28] have found that the odds ratio of experiencing a fall for community-dwelling older people taking one psychoactive medication was 1.5, while in those taking two or more of these drugs the odds ratio increased to 2.4.

Not all psychoactive medication subclasses are equally implicated in falls, however. The following section explores the evidence for the major psychoactive drug groups (hypnotics and anxiolytics, antidepressants and antipsychotics) as risk factors for falls.

Hypnotics and anxiolytics

The findings regarding the association between hypnotics and anxiolytics and falls are somewhat contradictory. Two case-control studies have reported no increased risk of falling for users of hypnotics and anxiolytics among older nursing home residents [21], and in a retrospective cohort community study, Prudham and Evans [29] found no difference in the use of hypnotics and anxiolytics between fallers and nonfallers. However, prospective studies have reported that hypnotics and anxiolytics carry a two- to fourfold increase in the risk of falling in institutionalized [11, 26, 30], and community-dwelling [31, 32] older people. To confuse matters further, there is some suggestion that, by reducing anxiety and depression, hypnotic and anxiolytic drugs may have beneficial effects in *preventing* falls [18]. These apparently discrepant results may be explained by differences in drug classification systems used in these studies [17], and by the finding that the actual dosage of the medication may be the important factor, rather than simply whether the drug is being taken or not [33].

When assessing the effects of hypnotics and anxiolytics, most studies explore the effects of benzodiazepines. These drugs are generally used for the treatment of anxiety and sleep disturbances [1]. Results regarding the specific subclass of benzodiazepines are more consistent, with several reporting a relationship between their use and increased falls risk [2, 33–36]. It has also been shown that the duration of use and gender may influence the extent of adverse outcomes. Neutel et al. [36] examined the relationship between the duration of benzodiazepine use and falls risk in older community residents, and reported that the greatest risk for falls injury was within 15 days of filling the prescription. With respect to gender differences, Trewin et al. [37] discovered that only lorazepam prescribed to women and nitrazepam prescribed to men were significantly associated with an increased falls risk, raising the possibility that males and females may have differing sensitivity to specific classes of benzodiazepines.

The differential effects of short- and long-acting benzodiazepines are unclear. Some studies have reported that long-acting benzodiazepines increase risk of falling [2, 38] and hip fracture [39] more so than short-acting drugs; however, other studies have found no significant differences between the two [21, 23]. An explanation for this discrepancy could be that dosage is more important than drug type. Recently, Herings et al. [33] reported that subjects taking more than the recommended dose had double the risk of hip fracture regardless of the actual type of benzodiazepine they had been prescribed.

Antidepressants

Antidepressants include the drug groupings of selective seratonin re-uptake inhibitors (SSRIs), tetracyclics, monamine oxidase inhibitors, and tricyclic antidepressants. The most commonly used antidepressants in long-term care facilities are SSRIs [40]. Evidence for the association between antidepressant use and falls risk seems to be divided with results both for [12, 16, 21, 30, 31, 34, 38, 41, 42] and against [2, 8, 11, 29]. These discrepant findings may be attributable, in part, to differing methodologies utilized. Overall, prospective designs have tended to report a significant association, whereas retrospective studies have not. The relationship between antidepressants and falls has been frequently observed even when controlling for variables such as medical conditions, dementia, functional status, age and body mass.

Specific classes of antidepressants and their effect on falls have also been investigated. Ray et al. [41] concluded that current users of tricyclic antidepressants had a significantly increased risk of hip fracture, while Ruthazer and Lipsitz [40] discovered that falls risk was greatest among women using SSRIs and tricyclic antidepressants. However, both Tinetti et al. [43] and Ebly et al. [16] found that no individual drug within the antidepressant group was clearly associated with falling. The significance of trends observed between different classes of antidepressants is limited by the small numbers of people taking these medications in the study samples.

Antipsychotics

Antipsychotics encapsulate a broad range of drug classes. Their primary objective is to reduce the symptoms of psychosis such as anxiety, acute agitation, hallucinations, delusions and delirium. In older people they are primarily prescribed to treat agitation in those with dementia. Work conducted among nursing home residents by Yip and Cumming [21] has found the most resounding support for the association between falls and antipsychotics. After adjusting for potential confounders, it was reported that residents using antipsychotic medications were four times more likely to fall than nonusers. This risk was also linearly related to increasing dosage. Similarly, case–control studies of hospitalized older people [44, 45] and nursing home residents [18, 26] have reported that the use of antipsychotic drugs is associated with a significant increased risk of experiencing an injurious fall. Whether this finding represents an inappropriate use of antipsychotics cannot be ascertained; however, it is interesting to note that one study has reported that the use of these drugs in patients with severe psychiatric illness actually *decreases* the risk of falling [46].

In contrast to the general consensus of antipsychotic drugs contributing to falls in long-term care facilities, studies involving community or intermediate care samples have generally not found antipsychotic drugs to be a risk factor for falls [2, 8, 38]. These findings can be interpreted in two ways. First, community dwellers using antipsychotic drugs may not comprise sufficient numbers to detect a significant relationship. Second, the predisposing effects of antipsychotics on falls may be more pronounced in long-term care residents where the prevalence of frailty, cognitive impairment and immobility are higher.

Pooling the data: meta-analysis findings for the relationship between psychoactive medications and falls

In a recently published systematic review, Leipzig et al. included data from much of the above literature in a meta-analysis to examine the relationship between psychoactive medications and falls in older people [47]. Significantly, only 40 studies were considered of a high enough quality to meet the authors' inclusion

Table 5.1. Pooled odds ratios for falling associated with psychoactive medication classes

Drug class	Number of studies	Pooled odds ratio
Sedatives / hypnotics	10	1.25 (0.98–1.60)
Benzodiazepines	8	1.40 (1.11–1.76)
Antipsychotics	9	1.90 (1.35–2.67)
Antidepressants	11	1.62 (1.23–2.14)
Tricyclic antidepressants	8	1.40 (0.96–2.02)
Any psychoactive medication	11	1.66 (1.40–1.97)

Source: Adapted from Leipzig et al. [47].

criteria, and none of these were randomized controlled trials. By pooling the odds ratios from the raw data of these studies, they found that psychotropic drugs were weakly but significantly associated with falls risk. These results are summarized in Table 5.1.

Cardiovascular system medications

Investigation of a relationship between cardiovascular medications and falls is meagre compared with studies exploring psychoactive medications and falls. Very few studies specifically explore cardiovascular medications, choosing instead to view them concurrently with other medications. Furthermore, there are problems associated with the classification of drugs studied. In some studies, diuretics are classified as antihypertensives, while other studies choose to investigate them as a separate entity. Results from studies that group cardiovascular classes into 'cardiac drugs' have been inconsistent [17]. The following cardiovascular medication groups: antihypertensive agents, diuretics and vasodilators/digoxin will each be considered in turn.

Antihypertensive agents

Angiotensin-converting enzyme (ACE) inhibitors, beta blockers and calcium channel blockers are the largest groups of antihypertensive drugs. These drugs are used in the management of angina pectoris and hypertension. There has been little support for an association between antihypertensives and falls. While some studies have reported that the use of antihypertensives is associated with a moderately increased risk of falling [8, 31, 32, 48] most studies have found a nonsignificant relationship for both older community [2, 29, 31, 34, 38, 49, 50] and long-term care residents [11, 51, 52]. The only prospective, randomized controlled trial on hypertensive use found no difference in falls prevalence between subjects taking the medication and those taking a placebo [53]. Given that the evidence for a relationship between the use of antihypertensive drugs and falling is weak, and that the risk of morbidity due to hypertension is high, it would appear that discontinuing the use of antihypertensive medications to prevent falls is not warranted in most cases [51].

Diuretics

Diuretics include drugs such as amiloride, thiazide and frusemide. These drugs are primarily used in the treatment of cardiac failure, hypertension, glaucoma and fluid retention. As with antihypertensives, there are few studies that report a significant relationship between the use of these medications and falls. While a small number of studies have found that fallers are more likely to be users of diuretics than nonfallers [2, 7], most studies fail to report any significance of diuretic use in terms of falls risk [4, 17, 20, 54]. Interestingly, there is some evidence that thiazide diuretics, by decreasing excretion of calcium in the urine, may have positive effects on bone density, thereby decreasing the risk of hip fracture [55].

Other cardiovascular system medications

Other cardiovascular medications that have come under investigation for their contributory role in falls risk include vasodilators and digoxin. Results are inconclusive, with some studies indicating a significant relationship [2, 30, 32, 35] and others showing no association [11, 14] between vasodilators and falls risk.

Digoxin is a cardiotonic drug used to strengthen weak heart muscle and to correct some forms of arrythmia. Gales and Mernard [23] reported that digoxin use increased falls risk in older people by 90% in an acute hospital setting, while a prospective study by Koski et al. [32] reported that the use of digoxin was associated with an increased risk of experiencing a fall-related minor injury for men, but not women. However, in each of these studies it is possible that the use of digoxin is simply a marker of physical frailty rather than a cause of falls.

Anti-inflammatories and analgesics

Anti-inflammatories include corticosteroids and nonsteroidal anti-inflammatory drugs (NSAIDs). These are primarily used to treat joint pain, stiffness, inflammation, gout and swelling associated with arthritis. Most epidemiological studies of anti-inflammatory medications and falls have only been concerned with NSAIDs. Results have again been mixed, with one report suggesting a relationship between NSAID use and falls in institutionalized older people [13], and others reporting no relationship [11, 38]. Interestingly, Yip and Cummings [21] found that while NSAID use did not reach statistical significance for two or more falls, it was an independent risk factor for four or more falls. This could be interpreted as suggesting that NSAIDs are only problematic for high-risk fallers; however, this finding needs to be treated with caution as the confounding variable of arthritis was not controlled for in the analysis. When the existence of arthritis is controlled for, odds ratios for falling are markedly reduced [2].

Narcotic analgesics (e.g. codeine and propoxyphene) have been found to produce psychomotor impairment, and in one study were significantly associated with hip fracture [56]. However, no relationship has been reported between narcotic analgesics and falls [23, 44]. The fundamental limitation in clarifying whether narcotics are related to falls is simply that there are only small numbers of older people taking these medications in the samples studied.

Pooling the data: meta-analysis findings for the relationship between cardiac and analgesic medications and falls

In the companion study to their work on psychoactive medications, Leipzig et al. conducted a systematic review and meta-analysis of the available research regarding cardiac and analgesic drugs [57] and falls in older people. As with the psychoactive review, only a minority of papers met the study's inclusion criteria, and again none were randomized controlled trials. By pooling the odds ratios from the raw data of these studies, it was concluded that digoxin, type IA antiarrythmic drugs are only weakly associated with falls risk, while no significant association was found for other cardiac drugs or analgesics. The results of this meta-analysis are summarized in Table 5.2.

Physiological mechanisms underlying the association between medications and falls

As indicated earlier, much of the research on medications and falls has focused on epidemiological designs establishing medications as falls risk factors, rather than delineating the possible mechanisms underlying the relationship. The complex nature of falls aetiology has made it difficult to make causal connections between medications and falls incidence. Knowledge of such issues may become somewhat clearer when investigations are undertaken on the physiological mechanisms by which certain medications predispose older persons to fall.

The main mechanism by which medications increase risk of falling may lie in the commonly encountered side effects they produce [58]. Reduced mental alertness, slowed transmission within the central nervous system, sedation, blurred vision, confusion, neuromuscular incoordination, impaired balance and drug-induced parkinsonism are all potential mechanisms by which some medications predispose older people to fall [20, 38].

Drug-induced postural hypotension may also be a potential contributor to falling. This is a common side effect of antidepressants, antipsychotics and diuretics/antihypertensives [21, 59]. In a large prospective study of community-dwelling

Table 5.2. Pooled odds ratios for falling associated with cardiac and analgesic medications

Drug class	Number of studies	Pooled odds ratio
NSAIDs	13	1.16 (0.97–1.38)
Aspirin	9	1.12 (0.80–1.57)
Nonnarcotic analgesics	9	1.09 (0.88–1.34)
Narcotic analgesics	13	0.97 (0.78–1.20)
Any diuretic	9	1.05 (0.96–1.14)
Thiazide diuretics	12	1.06 (0.97–1.16)
Loop diuretics	11	0.90 (0.73–1.12)
ACE inhibitors	10	1.20 (0.92–1.58)
Beta blockers	18	0.93 (0.77–1.11)
Calcium channel blockers	13	0.94 (0.77–1.14)
Centrally acting antihypertensives	11	1.16 (0.87–1.55)
Nitrates	14	1.13 (0.95–1.36)
Digoxin	17	1.22 (1.05–1.42)
Type 1a antiarrythmics	10	1.59 (1.02–2.48)

Notes:

NSAIDS, nonsteroidal anti-inflammatory drugs; ACE, angiotensin-converting enzyme.

Source: Adapted from Leipzig et al. [57].

women, we found a significant association between psychoactive medication use and postural hypotension [38]. However, evidence linking postural hypotension and falls is less convincing. While Davie et al. [6] found that systolic hypotension contributed independently to dizziness and falls, other studies have not reported such a relationship [38, 60, 61].

In addition to the potential impairments produced by medications in general, specific classes of drugs have been found to produce characteristic impairments in the sensory systems which contribute to balance and coordination. Benzodiazepines have been found to impair reaction time and increase postural sway in older people [59, 62–65], and an association has been reported between continuous benzodiazepine use and decreased position sense in the toes [59].

In a case–control study of factors associated with injurious falls, we have found associations between psychoactive medication use, quadriceps strength, and measures of standing balance [66], which suggests that benzodiazepines impair balance function both centrally and peripherally. Figure 5.1 shows a path analytic model for the relationship between psychoactive medication use and falls, derived from the Randwick falls and fractures study [38]. This analysis reveals that after adjusting for other interrelated and confounding factors (increased age, postural hypotension and inactivity), the association between psychoactive medication use and falls is

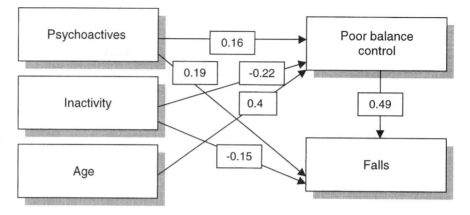

Fig. 5.1.   A path analytical model for the relationship between psychoactive medication use and falls. The standardized relative strengths of the effects (similar to correlation coefficients) are indicated by the numerals near the path arrows. This model indicates that, after adjusting for age and activity levels, approximately half of the association between psychoactive medication and falls is mediated via reduced stability. (Psychoactives: nil, one or two. Activity: hours per week. Age: age in years. Poor balance control: a composite measure incorporating measures of tactile sensitivity, vibration sense, quadriceps strength, reaction time, sway and clinical stability. Falls: two or more falls versus nil or one. Postural hypotension was found to be a statistically insignificant variable in the development of the final model.) Adapted from Lord et al. [38].

mediated, in large part, through poor balance control (as measured by a composite measure of sensory, motor, speed and stability variables). The remaining direct effect is likely to be due to other postulated side effects of these medications such as increased sedation and reduced mental alertness.

The mechanism by which NSAIDs may increase risk of falling is unclear, particularly given the problem of controlling for the confounding variable of osteoarthritis, itself a risk factor for falling [31, 67]. However, NSAIDs have been reported to produce central nervous system side effects such as impaired cognition, which may play a role in increasing falls risk [17].

Conclusion

Older people's use of and sensitivity to medications, combined with their susceptibility to fall, has ensured the importance of investigating the association between medications and falls. Most of the research to date has focused on the effects of psychoactive medication and falls risk in older people, and has found benzodiazepines, antipsychotic and antidepressant drugs to be significantly associated with increased falls risk. However, the relationship between antipsychotics and falls appears to be more pronounced for older residents in long-term care, and is likely to be confounded by the presence of dementia.

The research on cardiovascular medications is limited. There has been little support for an association between falls and various cardiac drugs such as anti-hypertensives. In addition, results indicate that nonsteroidal anti-inflammatories do not appear to be an independent risk factor for falls once the confounding variable of arthritis is taken into account.

Methodological limitations and the multifactorial nature of falls aetiology have made it difficult to make causal connections between medications and falls risk. Nevertheless, our knowledge of this complex issue is furthered by investigations exploring the physiological mechanisms by which certain medications or combinations of medications predispose older persons to fall. Physiological mechanisms purported to mediate the association between falls and medication use include changes in the central nervous system, postural hypotension, neuromuscular incoordination and impaired balance. Epidemiological research needs to be complemented by other forms of research focusing on psychomotor performance and fall-related parameters. In addition, further randomized controlled trials exploring the effects of interventions such as drug counselling and staged drug withdrawal need to be conducted.

REFERENCES

1 Jones D. Characteristics of elderly people taking psychotropic medication. *Drugs and Aging* 1992;2:389–94.
2 Cumming RG, Miller JP, Kelsey JL, et al. Medications and multiple falls in elderly people: the St Louis OASIS study. *Age and Ageing* 1991;20:455–61.
3 Macdonald JB. The role of drugs in falls in the elderly. *Clinics in Geriatric Medicine* 1985;1:621–36.
4 Chan DKY, Gibian T. Medications and falls in the elderly. *Australian Journal on Ageing* 1993;13:22–26.
5 Feely J, Coakley D. Altered pharmacodynamics in the elderly. *Clinics in Geriatric Medicine* 1990;6:269–83.
6 Davie JW, Blumenthal MD, Robinson-Hawkins S. A model of risk of falling for psychogeriatric patients. *Archives of General Psychiatry* 1981;38:463–7.
7 Sobel KG, McCart GM. Drug use and accidental falls in an intermediate care facility. *Drug Intelligence and Clinical Pharmacy* 1983;17:539–42.
8 Wells BG, Middleton B, Lawrence G, Lillard D, Safarik J. Factors associated with the elderly falling in intermediate care facilities. *Drug Intelligence and Clinical Pharmacy* 1985;19:142–5.
9 Campbell AJ, Borrie MJ, Spears GF. Risk factors for falls in a community-based prospective study of people 70 years and older. *Journal of Gerontology* 1989;44:M112–17.

10 Robbins AS, Rubenstein LZ, Josephson KR, Schulman BL, Osterweil D, Fine G. Predictors of falls among elderly people: results of two population-based studies. *Archives of Internal Medicine* 1989;149:1628–33.

11 Kerman M, Mulvihill M. The role of medication in falls among the elderly in a long-term care facility. *Mount Sinai Journal of Medicine* 1990;57:343–7.

12 Lipsitz LA, Jonsson PV, Kelley MM, Koestner JS. Causes and correlates of recurrent falls in ambulatory frail elderly. *Journal of Gerontology* 1991;46:M114–22.

13 Myers AH, Baker SP, Van Natta ML, Abbey H, Robinson EG. Risk factors associated with falls and injuries among elderly institutionalized persons. *American Journal of Epidemiology* 1991;133:1179–90.

14 Svensson ML, Rundgren A, Landahl S. Falls in 84- to 85-year-old people living at home. *Accident Analysis and Prevention* 1992;24:527–37.

15 Luukinen H, Koski K, Laippala P, Kivela SL. Risk factors for recurrent falls in the elderly in long-term institutional care. *Public Health* 1995;109:57–65.

16 Ebly EM, Hogan DB, Fung TS. Potential adverse outcomes of psychotropic and narcotic drug use in Canadian seniors. *Journal of Clinical Epidemiology* 1997;50:857–63.

17 Cumming RG. Epidemiology of medication-related falls and fractures in the elderly. *Drugs and Aging* 1998;12:43–53.

18 Nygaard HA. Falls and psychotropic drug consumption in long-term care residents: is there an obvious association? *Gerontology* 1998;44:46–50.

19 Cummings SR, Nevitt MC, Kidd S. Forgetting falls. The limited accuracy of recall of falls in the elderly. *Journal of the American Geriatrics Society* 1988;36:613–16.

20 Campbell AJ. Drug treatment as a cause of falls in old age. A review of the offending agents. *Drugs and Aging* 1991;1:289–302.

21 Yip YB, Cumming RG. The association between medications and falls in Australian nursing-home residents. *Medical Journal of Australia* 1994;160:14–18.

22 Thapa PB, Gideon P, Fought RL, Ray WA. Psychotropic drugs and risk of recurrent falls in ambulatory nursing home residents. *American Journal of Epidemiology* 1995;142:202–11.

23 Gales BJ, Menard SM. Relationship between the administration of selected medications and falls in hospitalized elderly patients. *Annals of Pharmacotherapy* 1995;29:354–8.

24 Luukinen H, Koski K, Laippala P, Kivela SL. Predictors for recurrent falls among the home-dwelling elderly. *Scandinavian Journal of Primary Health Care* 1995;13:294–9.

25 Mendelson WB. The use of sedative/hypnotic medication and its correlation with falling down in the hospital. *Sleep* 1996;19:698–701.

26 Mustard CA, Mayer T. Case–control study of exposure to medication and the risk of injurious falls requiring hospitalization among nursing home residents. *American Journal of Epidemiology* 1997;145:738–45.

27 Ray WA, Griffin MR, Schaffner W, Baugh DK, Melton LJD. Psychotropic drug use and the risk of hip fracture. *New England Journal of Medicine* 1987;316:363–9.

28 Weiner DK, Hanlon JT, Studenski SA. Effects of central nervous system polypharmacy on falls liability in community-dwelling elderly. *Gerontology* 1998;44:217–21.

29 Prudham D, Evans JG. Factors associated with falls in the elderly: a community study. *Age and Ageing* 1981;10:141–6.

30 Granek E, Baker SP, Abbey H, et al. Medications and diagnoses in relation to falls in a long-term care facility. *Journal of the American Geriatrics Society* 1987;35:503–11.

31 Blake A, Morgan K, Bendall M, et al. Falls by elderly people at home: prevalence and associated factors. *Age and Ageing* 1988;17:365–72.

32 Koski K, Luukinen H, Laippala P, Kivela SL. Physiological factors and medications as predictors of injurious falls by elderly people: a prospective population-based study. *Age and Ageing* 1996;25:29–38.

33 Herings RM, Stricker BH, de Boer A, Bakker A, Sturmans F. Benzodiazepines and the risk of falling leading to femur fractures. Dosage more important than elimination half-life. *Archives of Internal Medicine* 1995;155:1801–7.

34 Tinetti ME, Speechley M, Ginter SF. Risk factors for falls among elderly persons living in the community. *New England Journal of Medicine* 1988;319:1701–7.

35 Ryynanen OP, Kivela SL, Honkanen R, Laippala P, Saano V. Medications and chronic diseases as risk factors for falling injuries in the elderly. *Scandinavian Journal of Social Medicine* 1993;21:264–71.

36 Neutel CI, Hirdes JP, Maxwell CJ, Patten SB. New evidence on benzodiazepine use and falls: the time factor. *Age and Ageing* 1996;25:273–8.

37 Trewin VF, Lawrence CJ, Veitch GB. An investigation of the association of benzodiazepines and other hypnotics with the incidence of falls in the elderly. *Journal of Clinical Pharmacy and Therapeutics* 1992;17:129–33.

38 Lord SR, Anstey KJ, Williams P, Ward JA. Psychoactive medication use, sensori-motor function and falls in older women. *British Journal of Clinical Pharmacology* 1995;39:227–34.

39 Cumming RG, Klineberg RJ. Psychotropics, thiazide diuretics and hip fractures in the elderly. *Medical Journal of Australia* 1993;158:414–17.

40 Ruthazer R, Lipsitz LA. Antidepressants and falls among elderly people in long-term care. *American Journal of Public Health* 1993;83:746–9.

41 Ray WA, Griffin MR, Malcolm E. Cyclic antidepressants and the risk of hip fracture. *Archives of Internal Medicine* 1991;151:754–6.

42 Thapa PB, Gideon P, Cost TW, Milam AB, Ray WA. Antidepressants and the risk of falls among nursing home residents. *New England Journal of Medicine* 1998;339:875–82.

43 Tinetti ME, Williams TF, Mayewski R. Fall risk index for elderly patients based on number of chronic disabilities. *American Journal of Medicine* 1986;80:429–34.

44 Sorock GS. A case–control study of falling incidents among the hospitalized elderly. *Journal of Safety Research* 1983;14:47–52.

45 Mion LC, Gregor S, Buettner M, Chwirchak D, Lee O, Paras W. Falls in the rehabilitation setting: incidence and characteristics. *Rehabilitation Nursing* 1989;14:17–22.

46 Spar JE, LaRue A, Hewes C. Multivariate prediction of falls in elderly inpatients. *International Journal of Geriatric Psychiatry* 1987;2:185–8.

47 Leipzig RM, Cumming RG, Tinetti ME. Drugs and falls in older people: a systematic review and meta-analysis. I. Psychotropic drugs. *Journal of the American Geriatrics Society* 1999;47:30–9.

48 Lord SR, Ward JA, Williams P, Anstey KJ. Physiological factors associated with falls in older community-dwelling women. *Journal of the American Geriatrics Society* 1994;42:1110–17.

49 Perry BC. Falls among the elderly living in high-rise apartments. *Journal of Family Practice* 1982;14:1069–73.

50 O'Loughlin JL, Robitaille Y, Boivin JF, Suissa S. Incidence of and risk factors for falls and injurious falls among the community-dwelling elderly. *American Journal of Epidemiology* 1993;137:342–54.

51 Stegman MR. Falls among elderly hypertensives: are they iatrogenic? *Gerontology* 1983;29:399–406.

52 Maki BE, Holliday PJ, Topper AK. A prospective study of postural balance and risk of falling in an ambulatory and independent elderly population. *Journal of Gerontology* 1994;49:M72–84.

53 Curb JD, Applegate WB, Vogt TM. Antihypertensive therapy and falls and fractures in the systolic hypertension in the elderly program. *Journal of the American Geriatrics Society* 1993;41:SA15.

54 Cauley JA, Cummings SR, Seeley DG, et al. Effects of thiazide diuretic therapy on bone mass, fractures, and falls. The Study of Osteoporotic Fractures Research Group. *Annals of Internal Medicine* 1993;118:666–73.

55 Jones G, Nguyen T, Sambrook PN, Eisman JA. Thiazide diuretics and fractures: can meta-analysis help? *Journal of Bone and Mineral Research* 1995;10:106–11.

56 Schorr RI, Griffen MR, Daugherty JR. Opioid analgesics and the risk of hip fracture in the elderly: codeine and propoxyphene. *Journal of Gerontology* 1992;47:M111–15.

57 Leipzig RM, Cumming RG, Tinetti ME. Drugs and falls in older people: a systematic review and meta-analysis, II. Cardiac and analgesic drugs. *Journal of the American Geriatrics Society* 1999;47:40–50.

58 Sorock GS. Falls among the elderly. epidemiology and prevention. *American Journal of Preventive Medicine* 1988;4:282–8.

59 Sorock GS, Shimkin EE. Benzodiazepine sedatives and the risk of falling in a community-dwelling elderly cohort. *Archives of Internal Medicine* 1988;148:2441–4.

60 Ensrud KE, Nevitt MC, Yunis C, Hulley SB, Grimm RH, Cummings SR. Postural hypotension and postural dizziness in elderly women. The study of osteoporotic fractures. The Study of Osteoporotic Fractures Research Group. *Archives of Internal Medicine* 1992;152:1058–64.

61 Liu BA, Topper AK, Reeves RA, Gryfe C, Maki BE. Falls among older people: relationship to medication use and orthostatic hypotension. *Journal of the American Geriatrics Society* 1995;43:1141–5.

62 Swift CG, Ewen JM, Clarke P, Stevenson IH. Responsiveness to oral diazepam in the elderly: relationship to total and free plasma concentrations. *British Journal of Clinical Pharmacology* 1985;20:111–18.

63 Swift CG, Swift MR, Ankier SI, Pidgen A, Robinson J. Single dose pharmacokinetics and pharmacodynamics of oral loprazolam in the elderly. *British Journal of Clinical Pharmacology* 1985;20:119–28.

64 Robin DW, Hasan SS, Edeki T, Lichtenstein MJ, Shiavi RG, Wood AJ. Increased baseline sway contributes to increased losses of balance in older people following triazolam. *Journal of the American Geriatrics Society* 1996;44:300–4.

65 Liu YJ, Stagni G, Walden JG, Shepherd AMM, Lichtenstein MJ. Thioridazine dose-related

effects on biomechanical force platform measures of sway in young and old men. *Journal of the American Geriatrics Society* 1998;46:431–7.

66 Lord SR, McLean D, Stathers G. Physiological factors associated with injurious falls in older people living in the community. *Gerontology* 1992;38:338–46.

67 Dolinis J, Harrison JE, Andrews GR. Factors associated with falling in older Adelaide residents. *Australian and New Zealand Journal of Public Health* 1997;21:462–8.

6

Environmental risk factors for falls

Environmental factors have been said to contribute to falls for many years [1–3]. This chapter assesses the importance of a range of environmental factors in predicting falls. This involves discussion of the proportion of falls which may involve environmental factors, aspects of indoor and outdoor environments which have been suggested to contribute to falls, the strength of the evidence for the role of these factors in falling and the interaction between the environment and the older person's physical capabilities. Chapter 9 in the second part of this book will outline and examine the effectiveness of strategies to address potential environmental hazards.

Proportion of falls involving environmental factors

One method for assessing the contribution of various environmental factors to falling is to analyse the location and cause of falls. As discussed in Chapter 1, around half of all falls experienced by healthy community-dwellers occur within the person's own home [4–7]. Campbell et al. [6] found that 16% of falls occurred in the person's own garden, 21% in a bedroom, 19% in the kitchen and 27% in the lounge/dining room. Our group found 6% of falls occurred while using the shower or bath, 3% off a chair or ladder, 6% on stairs and 26% while walking on a level surface [7]. This indicates that many falls occur while the person is carrying out ordinary tasks. These figures also highlight the potential influence of environmental factors in gardens, public places and in other people's homes, in addition to those within the person's own home.

The location of falls varies for people of different ages and for men and women. With increasing age more falls occur inside the home on level surfaces [7]. Women are more likely to fall within their usual residence, while men are more likely to fall in their own garden [6]. Similarly, men are more likely to suffer a hip fracture outdoors [8].

In investigating the role of environmental risk factors we also need to consider the reported causes of falls. It would seem that falls related to trips and slips would be most likely to be related to environmental causes. Studies have found that between 21% [6] and 53% [7] of falls are attributed to these causes. While up to 14% of people are unable to identify the cause of their fall, 21% report losing their balance and 6% report their legs giving way [7]. These falls seem to be primarily 'intrinsic' (caused by factors within the person such as decreased muscle strength and poor balance) rather than 'extrinsic' (caused by external factors).

Some investigators have asked fallers directly whether the fall was associated with an environmental factor. Among community-dwellers this figure has been reported to be around 45% [5, 9, 10]. The role of environmental factors is less clear for falls causing a hip fracture. One study [11] found that 25% of these falls were associated with an environmental hazard, while another found this figure to be 58% [12]. These differences are probably due to variations in definitions and coding procedures. Therefore, environmental factors seem to play an important but not exclusive role in falling.

Suggested environmental risk factors

A number of authors have suggested that various environmental risk factors are associated with falling. These factors are usually identified from reports of fallers and observation of environments [3, 11, 13–21]. Posited environmental risk factors for falling are summarized in Table 6.1. Suggested measures to address each risk factor are outlined in Table 9.1.

Evidence regarding environmental risk factors

Private residences

As with other risk factors, it should be remembered that stronger evidence about the importance of an environmental risk factor is provided from prospective cohort studies, which assess environmental factors first and then monitor fall rates over a period of time. The next best evidence comes from case–control studies which involve assessment of environmental hazards among people who have and have not fallen. Weaker evidence comes from surveys where authors ask people who have fallen whether environmental factors were involved [22].

Several prospective cohort studies have now been conducted in this area. One of these showed some association between environmental risk factors and falling [5]. This study involved 325 older people who had suffered a fall in the previous year. Subjects completed a take-home questionnaire to assess structural hazards, tripping and slipping hazards, safety awareness and habits, and environmental obstacles. A subset of 70 subjects also had a nurse practitioner survey their home using the same questionnaire. None of the individual items or composite scores were

Table 6.1. Posited environmental risk factors

General
Slippery floor surfaces
Loose rugs
Upended carpet edges
Raised door sills
Obstructed walkways
Cord across walkways
Shelves or cupboards too high or too low
Spilt liquids
Pets

Furniture
Low chairs
Low or elevated bed height
Unstable furniture
Use of ladders and step ladders

Bathroom/toilet/laundry
Lack of grab rails shower/ bathtub/ toilet
Hob on shower recess
Low toilet seat
Outdoor toilet
Slippery surfaces
Use of bath oils

Stairs
No or inadequate handrails
Noncontrasting steps
Stairs too steep, tread too narrow
Distracting surroundings
Unmodifiable stairs or individual unable to manage stairs

Outdoors
Sloping, slippery, obstructed or uneven pathways, ramps and stairways
Brief cycles in traffic lights
Crowds
Certain weather conditions (leaves, snow, ice, rain)
Lack of places to rest
Unsafe garbage bin use

significantly associated with the risk of falls during the one-year study period. However, there was an increased risk of multiple falls among people who reported that one or more environmental factors (such as poor lighting or low seats) interfered with their ability to carry out activities of daily living in the home. This association remained significant after multivariate adjustment for a number of other variables. This implies that the role of the environment was more important in those with particular physical disabilities.

From the same study, Northridge et al. [23] classified subjects as either vigorous or frail. Not surprisingly, they found that the frail group suffered more frequent falls. However, they also found that, while there was no effect of environmental hazards on fall rates among frail people, there was some indication that vigorous people living with more environmental hazards were more likely to fall. For this group, a four-point increase on a seven-point composite home hazard scale was associated with a threefold increase in the odds of falling. This suggests that the role of environmental factors is less important among frailer people. While this seems to be counter-intuitive, it is probably the case that frailer people (who are likely to be weaker and have poorer balance) are more likely to fall regardless of environmental factors. In contrast, particular hazards are required for more vigorous people to fall.

Three other large prospective cohort studies have failed to show a clear relationship between environmental risk factors and falling. Two of these studies involved a home assessment by a health professional. Tinetti et al. [10] conducted a cohort study of 336 people aged 75 and older. A home assessment was conducted by the nurse-researcher at baseline using a standardized 30-point checklist to identify hazards such as obstacles and poor lighting. The number of environmental hazards identified was not significantly associated with falling. However, further analysis of the data also revealed a similar finding to that made by Northridge et al. [23], that is, vigorous older people were more likely to have a fall associated with an environmental hazard (53%) than either transitional (36%), or frail (29%) people [24].

Campbell et al. [6] conducted a 12-month prospective study of falling among 761 people aged 70 and older. An occupational therapist conducted a home assessment at baseline. During the follow-up period, the majority of trip and slip falls occurred over normal household objects in an uncluttered environment. These objects had not been identified as hazards. The authors concluded that generalized home hazard assessment and modification is not appropriate as a public health measure, but may have a role to play among people with a disability. Although this recommendation appears to be inconsistent with the findings of Northridge et al. [23] and Speechley et al. [24], it may be that as well as having a greater relative importance among vigorous people who fall less frequently, environmental factors are also important in people with particular disabilities (such as following amputation or stroke) who require particular environmental modifications to function independently and safely.

The third study [25] involved a telephone interview to identify two commonly suggested home hazards: the presence of loose rugs and the absence of non-slip strips in the bath or shower. Neither of these factors was predictive of falling in 586 subjects assessed 1 year later.

None of three recent case–control studies, which have compared the homes of fallers with those of nonfallers, have found extensive associations between environmental hazards and falling. Sattin et al. [26] conducted standardized assessments of the homes of 270 older people who had recently sought treatment for fall-related injuries, and 691 sex- and age-matched control subjects. They did not find significantly more hazards among the fallers. In fact, a commonly postulated hazard, the presence of throw rugs, was associated with a decreased risk of an injurious fall (except among those aged 85 and older).

In a case–control study, McLean and Lord [27] assessed the homes of 50 older people who had recently been admitted to hospital as a result of a fall and 45 age- and sex-matched community-living nonfallers. Fallers were further distinguished on the basis of whether they fell in the home or outside. Home hazard scores did not differ between home fallers, outside fallers and nonfallers.

The homes of older people who had been referred to an occupational therapist were assessed for hazards by Clemson et al. [28]. Subjects were 52 people with a recent hip fracture, 43 fallers and 157 nonfallers. The results indicated that the homes of fallers were no more hazardous than the homes of non-fallers. However, it was found that fallers with a cognitive impairment had more home hazards than fallers with no cognitive impairments and that a wide range of hazards was associated with hip fractures. Although the authors suggest that these results be interpreted carefully (as the assessors were not blind to fracture status), they highlight the need for further investigation of the relationship between home hazards and fractures.

Tinetti et al. [29] present further evidence of the relationship between environmental factors and the extent of injury suffered. From a nested cohort study they report that of 568 people who fell in a 36-month period, 69 suffered a serious injury (defined as a fracture, joint dislocation or head injury) during their first reported fall. A fall on stairs was independently associated with suffering a twofold increased risk of serious injury.

Temporary hazards and hazards within other people's homes may also contribute to falls. However, neither of these will be identified in studies involving home assessment. After conducting in-depth interviews with 15 people who had fallen, Connell and Wolf [30] found that temporary hazards played a role in a number of these falls. In addition, people may actually be more at risk from environmental hazards in other people's homes, as they may be unfamiliar with potential hazards, whereas in their own homes they may be better able to avoid them.

Residential aged care facilities

Residents of aged care facilities (hostels and nursing homes) are generally frailer than those living in private homes. It is therefore likely that in these settings, the person's physical impairments will play a relatively greater role in their risk of falling. In other words, these people may fall in the absence of any environmental hazard. In addition, these environments are often designed to minimize environmental hazards (e.g. absence of steps, wide corridors, presence of grab rails). Despite this, falls in residential care settings have also been found to involve environmental hazards. Therefore, even among frailer people, some falls have the potential to be prevented by environmental interventions.

Fleming and Pendergast [31] surveyed 294 fall incident reports for 95 residents of an adult care facility and found that 50% of the descriptions implicated an environmental factor, with pieces of furniture being the most common, followed by walking aids. Fifty-seven per cent of falls occurred in the residents' rooms. Similarly, Tinetti et al. [32] found that of 25 recurrent fallers, no falls were entirely explained by an environmental hazard. However, at least one fall for 23 of the 25 incidents involved an object (e.g. missing a chair while sitting down, falling while getting off the toilet). In a detailed review of falls in a nursing home setting, Rubenstein et al. [33] note that continence problems have been suggested to play an important role in nursing home falls, due to the need for repeated visits to the toilet during the day and at night. He suggests that environmental factors contributing to this problem are wet floors due to incontinence, poor lighting, bedrails and inappropriate bed height.

While recently built residential aged care facilities should be designed to maximize safety, it also seems to be important that the environment is well adapted to the individual (i.e. correct bed and chair heights) and that obvious risks (such as wet floors and clutter) are minimized [18, 33].

Public places

The issue of falls in public places is a vital one for public authorities. Over 10 000 claims for compensation for injuries sustained as a direct result of tripping over broken, uneven, or loose paving stones are made against local authorities in England and Wales annually [34]. Despite this, the issue of environmental risk factors in public places has been given little attention in the literature.

Reports from fallers indicate that environmental factors may have a greater role to play in outdoor falls than in indoor falls. Nevitt et al. [5] report that environmental factors (stairs or tripping and slipping hazards) were associated with 61%

of falls that occurred away from home and 33% of those that occurred at home. Norton et al. [11] report similar results for those who have suffered a hip fracture: environmental hazards were involved in 25% of falls at home, and in 56% of falls occurring away from home. In a study of 237 Accident and Emergency patients who had fallen in public places, two-thirds fell on pavements, 11% when crossing the road and 9% in shops [35].

The STEPS project [36] was a participatory research project where people were encouraged to report falls in public places to a telephone hotline. Of the 533 callers, 35% had some type of physical disability. Eighty-five per cent of incidents (falls and missteps) were in outdoor locations and the majority were on the footpath (sidewalk), an uneven surface or on a concrete surface. The authors call for ongoing community monitoring of falls hazards.

It is likely that the type of surface on which one falls affects the chance of suffering an injury. In their prospective study [37], Nevitt et al. report trends indicating an increased risk of injury with falls on hard surfaces such as pavement or concrete, but note than an earlier study [38] failed to find such an association. In a later case–control study, Nevitt and Cummings [39] found the risk of hip fracture to be significantly increased with falls on hard surfaces. However, two other case–control studies have not found such an association [40, 41].

The interaction between the individual and the environment

While it is evident from the studies outlined above that environmental factors are not the major cause of the majority of falls, interaction between an environmental hazard (or extrinsic factor) and the person's physical abilities (intrinsic factors) seems to play an important role in falls. Lawton [42] describes a model of the interaction between an older person's competence and the demands of the environment. A person must have a high competence level to cope effectively in an environment with high demands, while a person with a low competence level will be able to cope with an environment with low demands. As shown in Figure 6.1, we have adapted this model to describe the interaction between physical ability, environmental demand and the resultant risk of falling. Those with high physical abilities can withstand a range of environmental challenges without falling, yet when faced with an extreme challenge (e.g. a patch of ice) they may still fall. Those with lower physical abilities can generally cope well in an environment that offers few challenges (e.g. by staying indoors), yet when these abilities are very poor, a fall will be experienced regardless of the safety of the environment (e.g. a fall while walking on a level surface in a bathroom with rails installed). For example, if a more able person trips on a cracked footpath, they may have the ability to recover from this and avoid a fall. Yet a person with impairments in proprioception, reaction

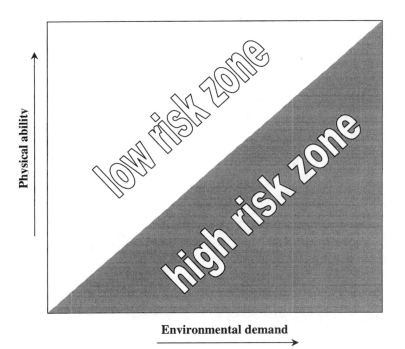

Fig. 6.1   Interaction between physical ability and environmental demand. The shaded area
represents an increased risk of falling.

time and/or muscle strength may not be able to recover in this way. This model is
helpful in understanding the findings of studies outlined above. The frail people
described by Northridge et al. [23] were probably falling in large part regardless of
their environment, while the more vigorous people fell when challenged by the
environment, thus environmental hazards played a more important role in their
falls.

Results reported by several other authors are consistent with this model. In a
study of over 1400 community-dwellers, Weinberg and Strain [43] found that those
with better self-rated health and those falling outdoors were more likely to attribute this fall to the surroundings. Those with poorer self-rated health and those who
reported having dexterity difficulties were more likely to attribute their falls to their
own limitations.

Studenski et al. [44] used a mobility screen to classify 306 people aged 70 years
and older as being at low (immobile, or mobile and stable) or high (mobile and
unstable) risk of falling. Being classified as high risk was strongly predictive of experiencing recurrent falls during the 6-month follow-up period. Among those
classified as high risk, an elevated risk score on a standardized environmental home
assessment was predictive of recurrent falls. A 10-point increase in environmental
risk score (out of a total 100) was associated with a 23% increase in fall risk. It seems

that those at low risk of falling were either better able to withstand environmental challenges or were not as challenged by their environments as the high-risk people.

The type of environmental challenges that an older person chooses to expose themself to, or in other words, the extent of a person's risk-taking behaviour would be expected to be an important part of the interaction between the person and their environment. Indeed, a person's attitude to risk (on a three-point scale) has been found to be associated with increased falls [44].

Conclusion

Identifiable environmental hazards have not been found to be major risk factors for falling among older people as a whole. This is particularly the case for older people's own homes. However, the interaction between an older person's physical abilities and exposure to environmental stressors does appear to be central to their risk of falling. Although falling rates are lower in vigorous older people than in their frailer counterparts, environmental hazards have a higher contribution to falls in this group. This appears to be due to increased exposure to higher risk activities as well as environments. There is also some evidence that the type of surface on which an older person falls affects the chance of suffering an injury.

REFERENCES

1 Castle O. Accidents in the home. *Lancet* 1950;1:315–19.

2 Droller H. Falls among elderly people living at home. *Geriatrics* 1955;10:239–44.

3 Sattin RW. Falls among older persons: a public health perspective. *Annual Review of Public Health* 1992;13:489–508.

4 Blake AJ, Morgan K, Bendall MJ, et al. Falls by elderly people at home: prevalence and associated factors. *Age and Ageing* 1988;17:365–72.

5 Nevitt MC, Cummings SR, Kidd S, Black D. Risk factors for recurrent nonsyncopal falls. A prospective study. *Journal of the American Medical Association* 1989;261:2663–8.

6 Campbell AJ, Borrie MJ, Spears GF, Jackson SL, Brown JS, Fitzgerald JL. Circumstances and consequences of falls experienced by a community population 70 years and over during a prospective study. *Age and Ageing* 1990;19:136–41.

7 Lord SR, Ward JA, Williams P, Anstey KJ. An epidemiological study of falls in older community-dwelling women: the Randwick falls and fractures study. *Australian Journal of Public Health* 1993;17:240–5.

8 Allander E, Gullberg B, Johnell O, Kanis JA, Ranstam J, Elffors L. Falls and hip fracture. A reasonable basis for possibilities for prevention? Some preliminary data from the MEDOS study; (Mediterranean osteoporosis study). *Scandinavian Journal of Rheumatology* 1996;103:49–52.

9 Morfitt JM. Falls in old people at home: intrinsic versus environmental factors in causation. *Public Health* 1983;97:115–20.

10 Tinetti ME, Speechley M, Ginter SF. Risk factors for falls among elderly persons living in the community. *New England Journal of Medicine* 1988;319:1701–7.

11 Norton R, Campbell AJ, Lee-Joe T, Robinson E, Butler M. Circumstances of falls resulting in hip fractures among older people. *Journal of the American Geriatrics Society* 1997;45:1108–12.

12 Parker MJ, Twemlow TR, Pryor GA. Environmental hazards and hip fractures. *Age and Ageing* 1996;25:322–5.

13 Archea JC. Environmental factors associated with stair accidents by the elderly. *Clinics in Geriatric Medicine* 1985;1:555–69.

14 Gibson MJ, Andres RO, Isaacs B, Radebaugh T, Worm-Petersen J. The prevention of falls in later life. A report of the Kellogg International Work Group on the prevention of falls by the elderly. *Danish Medical Bulletin* 1987;34:1–24.

15 Sjogren H, Bjornstig U. Injuries to the elderly in the traffic environment. *Accident Analysis and Prevention* 1991;23:77–86.

16 Clemson L, Roland M, Cumming R. Occupational therapy assessment of potential hazards in the homes of elderly people: an inter-rater reliability study. *Australian Occupational Therapy Journal* 1992;39:23–6.

17 Hemenway D, Solnick SJ, Koeck C, Kytir J. The incidence of stairway injuries in Austria. *Accident Analysis and Prevention* 1994;26:675–9.

18 Connell BR. Role of the environment in falls prevention. *Clinics in Geriatric Medicine* 1996;12:859–80.

19 Ryan JW, Spellbring AM. Implementing strategies to decrease risk of falls in older women. *Journal of Gerontological Nursing* 1996;22:25–31.

20 Tideiksaar R. Preventing falls: how to identify risk factors, reduce complications. *Geriatrics* 1996;51:43–55.

21 Carter SE, Campbell EM, Sanson-Fisher RW, Redman S, Gillespie WJ. Environmental hazards in the homes of older people. *Age and Ageing* 1997;26:195–202.

22 Hennekens C, Buring J. *Epidemiology in medicine.* Boston: Little, Brown, 1987.

23 Northridge ME, Nevitt MC, Kelsey JL, Link B. Home hazards and falls in the elderly: the role of health and functional status. *American Journal of Public Health* 1995;85:509–15.

24 Speechley M, Tinetti M. Falls and injuries in frail and vigorous community elderly persons. *Journal of the American Geriatrics Society* 1991;39:46–52.

25 Teno J, Kiel DP, Mor V. Multiple stumbles: a risk factor for falls in community-dwelling elderly. A prospective study. *Journal of the American Geriatrics Society* 1990;38:1321–5.

26 Sattin RW, Rodriguez JG, DeVito CA, Wingo PA. Home environmental hazards and the risk of fall injury events among community-dwelling older persons. Study to Assess Falls Among the Elderly (SAFE) Group. *Journal of the American Geriatrics Society* 1998;46:669–76.

27 McLean D, Lord S. Falling in older people at home: transfer limitations and environmental risk factors. *Australian Occupational Therapy Journal* 1996;43:13–18.

28 Clemson L, Cumming RG, Roland M. Case–control study of hazards in the home and risk of falls and hip fractures. *Age and Ageing* 1996;25:97–101.

29 Tinetti ME, Doucette JT, Claus EB. The contribution of predisposing and situational risk factors to serious fall injuries. *Journal of the American Geriatrics Society* 1995;43:1207–13.

30 Connell BR, Wolf SL. Environmental and behavioral circumstances associated with falls at

home among healthy elderly individuals. Atlanta FICSIT Group. *Archives of Physical Medicine and Rehabilitation* 1997;78:179–86.

31 Fleming BE, Pendergast DR. Physical condition, activity pattern, and environment as factors in falls by adult care facility residents. *Archives of Physical Medicine and Rehabilitation* 1993;74:627–30.

32 Tinetti ME, Williams TF, Mayewski R. Fall risk index for elderly patients based on number of chronic disabilities. *American Journal of Medicine* 1986;80:429–34.

33 Rubenstein LZ, Josephson KR, Osterweil D. Falls and fall prevention in the nursing home. *Clinics in Geriatric Medicine* 1996;12:881–902.

34 David H, Freedman L. Injuries caused by tripping over paving stones: an unappreciated problem. *British Medical Journal* 1990;300:784–5.

35 Fothergill J, O'Driscoll D, Hashemi K. The role of environmental factors in causing injury through falls in public places. *Ergonomics* 1995;38:220–3.

36 Gallagher EM, Scott VJ. The STEPS project: participatory action research to reduce falls in public places among seniors and persons with disabilities. *Canadian Journal of Public Health. Revue Canadienne de Santé Publique* 1997;88:129–33.

37 Nevitt MC, Cummings SR, Hudes ES. Risk factors for injurious falls: a prospective study. *Journal of Gerontology* 1991;46:M164–70.

38 Waller J. Falls among the elderly: human and environmental factors. *Accident Analysis and Prevention* 1978;10:21–33.

39 Nevitt MC, Cummings SR. Type of fall and risk of hip and wrist fractures: the study of osteoporotic fractures. The Study of Osteoporotic Fractures Research Group. *Journal of the American Geriatrics Society* 1993;41:1226–34.

40 Grisso JA, Kelsey JL, Strom BL, et al. Risk factors for falls as a cause of hip fracture in women. The Northeast Hip Fracture Study Group. *New England Journal of Medicine* 1991;324:1326–31.

41 Cumming RG, Klineberg RJ. Fall frequency and characteristics and the risk of hip fractures. *Journal of the American Geriatrics Society* 1994;42:774–8.

42 Lawton M. *Environment and aging.* Monterey, CA: Brooks Cole, 1980.

43 Weinberg LE, Strain LA. Community-dwelling older adults' attributions about falls. *Archives of Physical Medicine and Rehabilitation* 1995;76:955–60.

44 Studenski S, Duncan PW, Chandler J, et al. Predicting falls: the role of mobility and nonphysical factors. *Journal of the American Geriatrics Society* 1994;42:297–302.

7

The relative importance of falls risk factors: an evidence-based summary

In this chapter, we have pooled the findings from published studies on falls risk factors reviewed in Chapters 1 to 6. However, rather than simply listing the many and varied psychosocial, demographic, physiological, health and environmental factors that have been posited as important falls risk factors, we have rated each factor according to the strength of the published evidence for each factor actually being associated with falls. To do this we have using the following star rating system:

*** strong evidence (consistently found in good studies),

** moderate evidence (usually but not always found),

* weak evidence (occasionally but not usually found) and

– little or no evidence (not found in published studies despite research to examine the issue).

The factors have been classified into areas that were covered in turn by the first six chapters from Part 1 of this book: psychosocial and demographic factors, postural stability factors, sensory and neuromuscular factors, medical factors, medication factors and environmental factors.

Psychosocial and demographic Factors

Table 7.1 shows that a number of psychosocial and demographic factors have been systematically studied as potential risk factors for falls. As falls are generally considered to be a marker of frailty and immobility it is not surprising that falls are associated with advanced age and activities of daily living (ADL) limitations. The finding that a history of falling is associated with future falls is also not surprising. Most studies undertaken in community settings have shown a higher incidence of falls in women. This may be due to reduced strength and increased visual field dependence in women [1]. In a recent study, our group has also found that older women are worse than older men in executing fast and accurate steps in a choice reaction stepping time task that required whole body movement [2]. However in hospitals and institutions, where the inpatient populations are subject to substantial selection biases (based on ill health, frailty, immobility, etc.), the reported

Table 7.1. Psychosocial and demographic factors associated with falls

Factor	Strength of association
Advanced age	***
Female gender	**
Living alone	**
History of falls	***
Inactivity	**
ADL limitations	***
Alcohol consumption	–

Notes:
*** Strong evidence; ** moderate evidence; * weak evidence; – no evidence. ADL, activities of daily living.

incidence of falling is similar for men and women. The finding that living alone is a risk factor for falls is most likely confounded by gender and by age, in that elderly women comprise the majority of this group.

As is described in Chapter 8, physical activity can improve strength, balance and functional abilities in older people [3] and can prevent falls [4]. However, being more physically active does not always prevent falls [5]. This is probably because the more physically active older person takes part in activities which increase exposure to falls risk situations. Clearly, this risk should be balanced against the benefits of increased physical functioning and independence that exercise brings.

The most surprising finding regarding associations between psychosocial factors and falls is that alcohol consumption has not been shown to be a falls risk factor. Despite examining the issue, no significant associations have been found between alcohol use and falls in several large-scale studies [6–11]. In fact, most of these studies have found that those who are current drinkers have fewer falls, than those who abstain [6, 7, 8, 10]. Campbell et al. [6] have suggested that this unexpected negative association may be due to alcohol use being lowest in those with poor physical health or those taking psychoactive drugs, although this was not the case in our community study [8]. It may also be the case that the lack of a positive association between alcohol use and falls is due to response and selection biases, in that heavy alcohol consumers may underreport their drinking levels or simply decline participation in research studies. However, despite the lack of an association between current alcohol use and falls, there is strong evidence that long-term high alcohol intake can lead to impaired health and cognitive impairment, and can exacerbate such conditions in older people [12].

Table 7.2. Balance and mobility factors associated with falls

Factor	Strength of association
Impaired stability when standing	**
Impaired stability when leaning and reaching	**
Inadequate responses to external perturbations	*
Slow voluntary stepping	**
Impaired gait and mobility	***
Impaired ability in standing up	***
Impaired ability with transfers	***

Notes:

*** Strong evidence; ** moderate evidence; * weak evidence; – no evidence.

Postural instability

Table 7.2 summarizes the results of the many investigations performed to assess whether various measures of postural stability are associated with increased falls risk. Generally speaking, the more challenging the stability task is, the stronger its evidence as a falls risk factor. For example, while impaired stability when standing and during leaning tasks are moderate risk factors, measures of gait, transfers and standing from a sitting position are consistently reported as strong risk factors in well-designed studies.

Although many studies have been performed to evaluate age-related differences in responding to platform perturbation, performance on these tests is only weakly associated with falls. There are two possible reasons for this. First, few large prospective studies have employed the mechanical perturbation model as it generally requires specialized equipment, and is therefore restricted to testing of smaller numbers of subjects in a balance laboratory. Second, the artificial perturbations induced by platform tests are quite dissimilar to those that would lead to a fall in an older person's daily environment. Interestingly, a recent prospective study by Maki et al. [13] found that while standing sway in the mediolateral direction predicted falls, performance on tests of mediolateral and anteroposterior platform perturbation were not able to discriminate between fallers and nonfallers. It would therefore appear that measures of postural stability will only be able to predict falls if the tests used challenge balance in a realistic manner that represents the context of the specific task being performed.

Table 7.3. Sensory and neuromuscular factors associated with falls

Factor	Strength of association
Visual acuity	**
Visual contrast sensitivity	***
Visual field dependence	*
Reduced peripheral sensation	***
Reduced vestibular function	–
Muscle weakness	***
Poor reaction time	***

Notes:
*** Strong evidence; ** moderate evidence; * weak evidence; – no evidence.

Sensory and neuromuscular factors associated with falls

As indicated in Chapter 3, there is general agreement that postural control is a complex process, which involves many body systems. Table 7.3 shows that reduced functioning in peripheral sensation, strength and reaction time – major contributors to balance control – are strongly associated with falls. Impaired vision is also likely to be a strong falls risk factor, and the fact that it has been found to be only moderately associated with falls appears to be due to the use of a suboptimal test, i.e. high-contrast letter charts. These charts measure discrimination of fine detail, whereas the detection of larger visual stimuli under low-contrast conditions has been found to be a more pertinent visual function for avoiding hazards and thus falls [14].

Vestibular function is the only physiological domain that has not been found to be associated with falls in older people. It may be that older people with adequate peripheral sensation and/or vision, can compensate for reduced vestibular functioning. However, as indicated in Chapter 3, the screening assessments used to measure vestibular function in the epidemiological studies of falls undertaken to date have been indirect and possibly too insensitive to be able to detect subtle yet significant impairments in vestibular function. Further research is required in this area.

In our studies, we have found that measurements of vision, peripheral sensation, strength, reaction time and balance significantly and independently contribute to the discrimination between fallers and nonfallers in multivariate analyses [15, 16]. This suggests that poor functioning in any of these physiological domains predisposes older people to falls, and that multiple impairments greatly increase falls risk. However, when the standardized weightings of each measure are compared, it is

Table 7.4. Medical factors associated with falls

Factor	Strength of association
Impaired cognition	***
Depression	**
Abnormal neurological signs	**
Stroke	***
Incontinence	**
Acute illness	**
Parkinson's disease	***
Vestibular disorders	–
Arthritis	**
Foot problems	**
Dizziness	*
Orthostatic hypotension	–

Notes:
*** Strong evidence; ** moderate evidence; * weak evidence;
– no evidence.

apparent that they do not contribute equally to the prediction of falls. Slow reaction time and increased sway (particularly when challenged by having subjects close their eyes or stand on a compliant surface) appear to be particularly strong physiological risk factors for falls [15, 16].

Medical factors

A number of researchers have now identified a range of medical factors that are associated with an increased risk of falls [6, 8–10, 17–20]. These include the presence of stroke or Parkinson's disease, acute illness, arthritis, foot problems, depression, impaired cognition, incontinence and abnormal neurological signs. These conditions have been shown to be risk factors for falls in both community and institutional settings, although the importance of some of these such as incontinence and impaired cognition (with associated antipsychotic drug use) may be more important in institutions. The distinction between strong and moderate evidence as indicated in Table 7.4 for these factors relates to some extent to the difficulty in rigorously measuring some of these conditions. This has meant that fewer studies have addressed these factors or that crude measures (with resultant imprecision) have been used as substitutes. This is particularly the case for neurological conditions, arthritis and foot problems. However, as also shown in Table 7.4, certain conditions commonly thought to be strong risk factors for falls, such as vestibular disorders and orthostatic hypotension, have not been found to be important risk factors in research studies.

The lack of reported associations between vestibular disorders and dizziness on the one hand and falls on the other appears paradoxical, as such disorders have marked effects on balance. Three factors could account for the lack of association. First, increased age results in a *loss* of vestibular functioning, not an increase in *aberrant* vestibular information, as is the case with vestibular disease. As indicated above, older people with adequate peripheral sensation and/or vision may be able to compensate for reduced vestibular functioning. Second, anecdotal evidence indicates that vestibular disorders (as opposed to diminished vestibular function) do have a marked effect on balance in older people, an effect that is patently clear to the sufferers and as a result they take steps to avoid falling – quite often by literally lying down. The final factor may relate to study limitations in that assessment measures for accurately measuring vestibular functioning have not been carried out in large prospective studies on falls.

As indicated in Chapter 4, orthostatic hypotension, whether idiopathic or due to a side effect of antihypertensive use, has not generally been found to increase the risk of falling in older people. This indicates that in comparison with impairments of sensorimotor function, balance and gait, orthostatic hypotension is a relatively unimportant or rare cause of falls. As is the case with vestibular disorders, the lack of a demonstrated link between orthostatic hypotension and falls may be due to study limitations. Most studies have tested for orthostatic hypotension on a single occasion, usually when the older subject visits a clinic or laboratory. These subjects are then followed up in prospective studies to determine falling rates. It is possible that as orthostatic hypotension can be of an intermittent nature, subjects may test negatively on the baseline testing day, but suffer postural blood pressure drops and falls on one or more occasions in the follow-up period.

Medication use

Table 7.5 outlines medications that have been implicated in falls in older people. Both community and institutional studies have consistently reported significant associations between falls and psychoactive and multiple drug use. Studies of non-steroidal anti-inflammatory drug (NSAID) use indicate that this medication does not appear to be an independent risk factor for falls once the confounding variable of arthritis is taken into account.

In contrast with the few studies that have made direct assessments of orthostatic hypotension, many studies have examined antihypertensive use as a possible falls risk factor. Here the findings have been inconsistent and a recent meta-analysis

Table 7.5. Medication factors associated with falls

Factor	Strength of association
Psychoactive medication use	***
Antihypertensive use	*
NSAIDs	–
Use of more than 4 medications	***

Notes:
*** Strong evidence; ** moderate evidence; * weak evidence; –
no evidence. NSAIDS, nonsteroidal anti-inflammatory drugs.

Table 7.6. Environmental factors associated with falls

Factor	Strength of association
Poor footwear	*
Inappropriate spectacles	*
Home hazards	–
External hazards	–

Notes:
*** Strong evidence; ** moderate evidence; * weak
evidence; – no evidence.

of the available published data concluded that there was little support for an
association between antihypertensive use and falls [21].

Environmental factors

In contrast to psychosocial, demographic, medical and physiological factors, Table
7.6 shows there is little evidence that environmental factors are primary risk factors
for falling. For example, it has not been found that older people who live in hazardous homes have more falls than those who live in safe homes. The lack of
associations may reflect, at least in part, the difficulty of studying transient or intermittent risk factors. However, as many falls do involve environmental factors, it
seems that the interaction between the older person's physical abilities and the
environment is a crucial factor in determining whether a fall will occur.

Although no studies have reported direct relationships between poor footwear
or inappropriate spectacles and falls, both of these factors have been found to affect
important falls risk factors. For example, high-heeled shoes impair balance [22]

and bifocal spectacles impair depth perception and contrast sensitivity at critical distances required for detecting obstacles in the environment [23].

Conclusion

Many psychosocial and medical conditions and impairments of sensorimotor function, balance and gait have been shown in large epidemiological studies to be strongly associated with falls. The lack of significant associations for other posited risk factors may indicate that these are relatively unimportant causes of falls or that these issues have not been subject to appropriate study. The risk factors that are of an intermittent nature have been especially difficult to study.

The above summaries have listed risk factors in isolation and have used a simple classification scheme. Many of the risk factors are interrelated, as preliminary path analytical models have shown [24]. Further the intrinsic/extrinsic distinction is an oversimplification, and a better understanding of falls is usually obtained when taking a ecological perspective, that is, examining the person in association with environmental factors [25]. Finally, the above summaries, by definition, were based on findings from population studies. Clearly, in clinical practice many medical conditions and disorders in addition to those listed above as important risk factors may well be the cause of falls in individual patients and require investigation.

REFERENCES

1 Lord, SR, Sambrook PN, Gilbert C, Kelly PJ, Nguyen T, Webster IW, Eisman JA. Postural stability, falls and fractures in the elderly: results from the Dubbo osteoporosis epidemiology study. *Medical Journal of Australia* 1994;160:684–91.

2 Lord SR, Matters B, Corcoran J, Howland A, Fitzpatrick R. Choice reaction time stepping: a composite measure of falls risk in older people. *Gait and Posture* 1999;9:S29.

3 Buchner DM, Beresford SA, Larson EB, LaCroix AZ, Wagner EH. Effects of physical activity on health status in older adults. II. Intervention studies. *Annual Review of Public Health* 1992;13:469–88.

4 Province MA, Hadley EC, Hornbrook MC, et al. The effects of exercise on falls in elderly patients. A preplanned meta-analysis of the FICSIT trials. Frailty and injuries: cooperative studies of intervention techniques. *Journal of the American Medical Association* 1995;273:1341–7.

5 Studenski S, Duncan PW, Chandler J, et al. Predicting falls: the role of mobility and nonphysical factors. *Journal of the American Geriatrics Society* 1994;42:297–302.

6 Campbell AJ, Borrie MJ, Spears GF. Risk factors for falls in a community-based prospective study of people 70 years and older. *Journal of Gerontology* 1989;44:M112–17.

7 Nelson DE, Sattin RW, Langlois JA, DeVito CA, Stevens JA. Alcohol as a risk factor for fall

injury events among elderly persons living in the community. *Journal of the American Geriatrics Society* 1992;40:658–61.

8 Lord SR, Ward JA, Williams P, Anstey KJ. An epidemiological study of falls in older community-dwelling women: the Randwick falls and fractures study. *Australian Journal of Public Health* 1993;17:240–5.

9 Sheahan SL, Coons SJ, Robbins CA, Martin SS, Hendricks J, Latimer M. Psychoactive medication, alcohol use, and falls among older adults. *Journal of Behavioral Medicine* 1995;18:127–40.

10 Tinetti ME, Speechley M, Ginter SF. Risk factors for falls among elderly persons living in the community. *New England Medical Journal* 1988;319:1701–7.

11 Nevitt MC, Cummings SR, Kidd S, Black D. Risk factors for recurrent nonsyncopal falls. A prospective study. *Journal of the American Medical Association* 1989;261:2663–8.

12 Carlson JE. Alcohol use and falls (letter). *Journal of the American Geriatrics Society* 1993;41:346.

13 Maki BE, Holliday PJ, Topper AK. A prospective study of postural balance and risk of falling in an ambulatory and independent elderly population. *Journal of Gerontology* 1994;49;M72–84.

14 Lord SR, Clark RD, Webster IW. Visual acuity and contrast sensitivity in relation to falls in an elderly population. *Age and Ageing* 1991;20:175–81.

15 Lord SR, Clark RD, Webster IW. Physiological factors associated with falls in an elderly population. *Journal of the American Geriatrics Society* 1991;39:1194–200.

16 Lord SR, Ward JA, Williams P, Anstey K. Physiological factors associated with falls in older community-dwelling women. *Journal of the American Geriatrics Society* 1994;42:1110–17.

17 Blake AJ, Morgan K, Bendall MJ, et al. Falls by elderly people at home: prevalence and associated factors. *Age and Ageing* 1988;17:365–72.

18 Campbell AJ, Reinken J, Allan BC, Martinez GS. Falls in old age: a study of frequency and related clinical factors. *Age and Ageing* 1981;10:264–70.

19 Prudham D, Grimley Evans J. Factors associated with falls in the elderly: a community study. *Age and Ageing* 1981;10:141–6.

20 Robbins AS, Rubenstein LZ, Josephson KR. Predictors of falls among elderly people. Results of two population-based studies. *Archives of Internal Medicine* 1989;149:1628–33.

21 Leipzig RM, Cumming RG, Tinetti ME. Drugs and falls in older people: a systematic review and meta-analysis, II. Cardiac and analgesic drugs. *Journal of the American Geriatrics Society* 1999;47:40–50.

22 Lord SR, Bashford G. Shoe characteristics and balance in older women. *Journal of the American Geriatrics Society* 1996;44:429–33.

23 Lord SR, Howland AS, Dayhew J. Effect of bifocal spectacles on contrast sensitivity and depth perception in older people. Proceedings of the Australian Association of Gerontology Annual Conference, Sydney, 1999.

24 Lord SR, Anstey K, Williams P, Ward JA. Psychoactive medication use, sensori-motor function and falls in older women. *British Journal of Clinical Pharmacology* 1995;39: 227–34.

25 Hogue CC: Falls and mobility in later life: an ecological model. *Journal of the American Geriatrics Society* 1984;32:858–61.

Part II

Strategies for prevention

Overview: Falls prevention

Risk factors for falling have been described in detail in the first part of this book and summarized in Chapter 7. The identification of risk factors is the first step in falls prevention. It is then necessary to establish which risk factors are potentially modifiable, so that relevant and appropriate intervention strategies aimed at preventing falls can be designed, implemented and evaluated [1].

The table lists the falls risk factors which we rated as either 'strongly' or 'moderately' associated with falls in published studies in Chapter 7. In addition, we have included certain other risk factors that are likely to be important but have yet to be shown to be so due to methodological difficulties. The table shows the extent to which these risk factors are modifiable and suggests broad intervention strategies for each.

It is evident from the table that some important risk factors are not modifiable. Nevertheless, an understanding of the causes and predisposing factors of falls can provide information for targeting prevention strategies and awareness-raising programmes.

The table also shows that many falls risk factors have considerable potential for intervention. These strategies are described in the remainder of this book. Chapters 8 to 14 review the studies that have examined the effects of particular behavioural and/or environmental interventions. Chapter 15 evaluates the effectiveness of targeted multifaceted falls prevention programmes and Chapter 16 outlines a physiological profile assessment approach that enables intervention programmes to be individually tailored to those most at risk.

REFERENCE

1 Tinetti ME, Baker DI, Garrett PA, Gottschalk M, Koch ML, Horwitz RI: Yale FICSIT: risk factor abatement strategy for fall prevention. *Journal of the American Geriatrics Society* 1993; 41: 315–20.

Falls risk factors: ability to be modified and intervention strategies

Risk Factor	Able to be modified?	Intervention strategies
Advanced age	No	Discussion of increased risk
Female	No	Discussion of increased risk
Living alone	Possibly	Discussion of increased risk and possible change of living arrangements
Inactivity	Yes	Exercise, education
Activities of daily living (ADL) limitations	Yes	Exercise, motor training, use of aids, provision of assistance with ADL
History of falls	No	Discussion of increased risk
Medical factors	Possibly	Appropriate medical or surgical intervention
Medications	Possibly	Medication withdrawal, investigation of alternative strategies
Poor vision	Possibly	Use of appropriate spectacles, appropriate medical/surgical intervention, discussion of increased risk
Reduced peripheral sensation	No	Discussion of increased risk and compensatory strategies
Muscle weakness	Yes	Strength training
Poor reaction time	Yes	Exercise/training of fast, coordinated responses, e.g. exercise to music
Impaired balance	Yes	Exercise/training involving control of movements of centre of mass
Impaired gait	Yes	Exercise/training targeting causes, consider use of aids and appliances
Footwear	Yes	Advice re appropriate footwear
Environmental hazards (home, institution, public place)	Yes	Installation of safety features, correction/removal of hazards

8

Exercise interventions to prevent falls

Exercise has a major role to play in modifying key falls risk factors and preventing falls among older adults. There are, however, many different types of exercise, some of which are likely to result in greater reductions in falls risk than others. Therefore, health professionals can do better than merely suggest that older people should exercise. As Hadley [1] states 'telling an older person that "exercise" could help prevent falls is not much better than telling them that "antibiotics" could help cure an infection: although true, the advice would be much more useful if it were more specific' (p. 1382).

To optimize the prescription of exercise to prevent an older person falling, the health professional can assess the person's performance on key physical measures of falls risk. The most appropriate form of exercise to address individual deficits found can then be determined. Possible exercise settings can then be discussed with the client. A range of other factors may also need to be considered when deciding on the most appropriate exercise for an individual. Among these are: financial status, carer responsibilities, availability of transport and personal preferences.

This chapter aims to assist the health professional to prescribe exercise by outlining different exercise forms and settings for older people and summarizing the evidence for their effects on falls and fall risk factors.

Exercise and falls

For several years now, it has been clear that exercise among older people can modify key falls risk factors such as decreased muscle strength and poor balance. However, until very recently, there has not been the evidence that exercise can actually reduce the incidence of falls. This may be partly because large sample sizes are required to investigate the effect of exercise on falls incidence rates, and because many studies of exercise do not measure falls. However, a number of recent studies have found a reduction in falls rates with several different forms of exercise.

The FICSIT (frailty and injuries: cooperative studies of intervention techniques) trials recently conducted in the USA have provided crucial information. These seven independent randomized controlled trials included an exercise component for 10–36 weeks. The nature of this intervention varied between trials. The pre-planned meta-analysis [2] of all seven trials included a total of 2328 older people. The adjusted fall incidence ratio for the treatment arms including general exercise was 0.90 (95% confidence interval 0.81–0.99) and for those including balance training it was 0.83 (95% CI 0.70–0.98). In other words, the incidence of falls was probably reduced by about 10% in those undertaking any exercise and by about 17% in those undertaking balance exercise.

Two individual FICSIT trials also found an effect of exercise alone on falling. From their randomized clinical trial of Tai Chi, computerized balance training and education, Wolf et al. [3] reported that the rate of falls was substantially (47.5%) reduced in the subjects who had participated in the 15-week Tai Chi programme.

In the Seattle FICSIT study, Buchner et al. [4] found that among 105 older people with at least mild deficits in strength and balance, exercise had a protective effect on risk of falling (relative hazard = 0.53, 95% CI 0.30–0.91). This study was a randomized trial of supervised strength and/or endurance training (1-hour sessions, three per week, for 24–26 weeks), followed by self-supervised exercise. Interestingly, exercise did not actually reduce fall rates in the intervention group, rather, fall rates increased in the control group. It seems, as the authors suggest, that exercise played a role in preventing deterioration.

The Yale FICSIT study found targeted multifaceted interventions to reduce falls incidence significantly [5]. One of the interventions used was a home exercise programme. However, this study design makes it difficult to assess the effectiveness of exercise as an individual component.

Another recent study has also shown an effect of exercise on falling. A randomized controlled trial by Campbell et al. [6] in New Zealand showed a reduction in falls rate and falls injuries with a home exercise programme (among 232 women aged 80 and over). The home exercise programme was established in four visits from a physiotherapist, while the control group received the same number of social visits. The relative hazard for the first four falls in the exercise group compared with the control group was 0.61 (95% CI 0.52–0.90).

However, not all studies in this area have found that exercise prevents falls. The FICSIT meta-analysis [2] found that interventions classified as resistance, endurance or flexibility training did not significantly affect fall rates. The Cochrane Collaboration systematic review [7], which involved pooling data from four randomized controlled trials involving exercise alone, did not find a significant effect on fall rates. However, as this review did not include two of the more recent studies outlined above, this conclusion may well be changed when the review is next updated.

Exercise options, falls and falls risk factors

There is ample evidence from many studies for the positive effects of various forms of exercise on key falls risk factors and functional abilities among older people. In this section, various forms of exercise will be discussed in terms of their background, effects on falls and falls risk and effects on functional abilities. In the background section, the aims, methods and prescription principles of each exercise intervention will be briefly outlined. The falls and falls risk section will consist of an overview of the results of randomized controlled trials investigating the effect of the particular exercise on falls incidence and on key risk factors for falls (such as strength, balance and gait). The functional abilities section will discuss the demonstrated and postulated effects of the intervention on an individual's ability to perform tasks central to independent daily living. As discussed previously, many measures of falls risk are also a reflection of the person's functional abilities. The final section of this chapter considers where exercise can be undertaken and the advantages and disadvantages of different settings.

Resistance training

Background

Resistance training aims to increase the ability of a muscle or group of muscles to generate force. It is based on the overload principle first described by Roux and Lange in the early twentiethth century, who suggested that performance of work of an intensity beyond its accustomed load would cause a muscle to grow in size and strength [8]. Progressive resistance training regimes for a range of patient groups were described by DeLorme and Watkins in the 1940s and 1950s [9]. Patients performed three sets of 10 repetitions at increasing proportions of a weight that could only be lifted 10 times (10 repetition maximum or 10RM), with the last set being at a 10RM intensity. In DeLorme's protocol, the 10RM was assessed weekly so that as the person became stronger, the load lifted was increased.

While the popular perception of resistance training continues largely to involve muscle-bound sweaty young men, a large number of controlled trials have now found resistance training to be safe and effective among older adults [10]. Several popular books aimed at older people outline practical aspects of strength training programmes for this age group [11, 12].

The American College of Sports Medicine [13] recommends that healthy sedentary adults undertake a strength training programme involving one set of 8–12RM of 8–10 different exercises twice weekly. It also recommends that older adults and people with cardiac disease carry out similar programmes at a slightly lower intensity (10–15RM) to decrease the risk of musculoskeletal injury and cardiac complications [14, 15]. While few studies have compared strength training at different intensities for older people, there is some evidence for a greater relative effectiveness of lower-intensity programmes compared with higher-intensity programmes than in younger people [16, 17]. To decrease the risk of injury, it is common for strength training programmes for older people to include a warm-up set at a lower intensity [10].

Older people with various medical conditions may still be able to benefit from a strength training programme. For example, resistance training has been shown to reduce physical disability and pain among older people with osteoarthritis [18]. High-intensity strength training (80% of 1RM) has been found to be safe and effective among aerobically trained cardiac patients [19].

However, the risk of a cardiovascular event occurring during exercise is substantially increased among those with cardiac disease. Guidelines published by the American College of Sports Medicine (ACSM) and the American Heart Association (AHA) [20] suggest that cardiovascular screening be undertaken before a person of any age commences a moderate to high intensity exercise programme. Two screening tools are suggested, the Revised *Physical activity readiness questionnaire* (PAR-Q) and the AHA/ACSM *Health/fitness facility preparticipation screening questionnaire.* If potential risk is identified on these brief questionnaires, the person is advised to contact their doctor for possible further investigation. These people should also exercise in a setting where medical or professional supervision is available.

Effects on falls and falls risk

Epidemiological studies have shown that muscle strength decreases with increased age [21], and that reduced muscle strength is one of the major risk factors for falling [22, 23]. Exercise interventions aimed at improving muscle strength have been widely identified as a key strategy for reducing frailty [24] and maintaining function [15] in old age.

It is now clear from a number of randomized controlled trials that resistance training can substantially increase muscle strength among community-dwelling older people [4, 25–31]. A typical programme would involve the person lifting a weight of 50–80% of their 1RM (the weight they are able to lift only once) using an exercise machine, two or three times weekly.

Resistance-training programmes have also been investigated among people living in supported accommodation. In a randomized controlled trial of a 10-week resistance exercise programme among 100 frail nursing home residents, Fiatarone et al. [32] demonstrated significant increases in muscle strength, gait velocity, stair-climbing power and level of spontaneous physical activity in the exercisers compared with the controls. Several other noncontrolled studies have also demonstrated the feasibility of this type of approach among nursing home residents [33, 34].

Effects on functional abilities

While some authors argue that improved strength in older people will result in augmented functional ability [15], other evidence suggests that this may not necessarily be the case.

It has been found that a nonlinear relationship exists between strength and function among older people [35]. Buchner et al. reported than among weaker people, leg strength and gait speed were associated, whereas among stronger people there was no relationship between the variables. It appears that the stronger people were able to generate sufficient levels of muscle tension to successfully carry out the task, while the weaker people's lack of strength impaired performance of the task [35]. The level of strength required for a particular task has been referred to as the threshold value [36]. Threshold values have been identified for various tasks [37–39].

It seems likely that for people below this critical level of strength, strength training will lead to improved functional abilities [40]. However, among stronger people (who already have sufficient strength for functional tasks), an increase in strength will not improve functional performance.

Studies among younger people have shown that the greatest improvements in muscle strength occur for the muscle action which has been trained and that carry-over to other muscle actions is limited [8, 41]. This principle of specificity of training has been shown to apply to the task trained [42], the velocity of contractions [43], and the angle of isometric contractions [44]. This means that strength training for isolated muscle groups in positions and velocities not relevant to the everyday tasks may not be the most effective way to increase functional ability. In other words, seated resistance training may improve the ability to lift a weight using the quadriceps muscle in sitting, but may not improve stair-climbing ability. As Rutherford [45] suggests 'rather than using conventional exercises to strengthen individual muscle groups it may be more advantageous to identify particular functional deficits and then repeatedly practise these with or without added resistance' (p. 201). While this approach is yet to be investigated among older people it seems that task-related resistance training could have a greater effect on functional abilities than more traditional nonweight-bearing resistance training.

Unfortunately, many strength training studies do not measure functional abilities so do not offer additional information on this question. Several studies of nonweight-bearing strength training have not shown any improvement in functional ability [4, 46] or have shown improvement on only one or two of a number of functional measures [31, 47]. Two studies have shown improved functional abilities with strength training for very high level tasks (backward tandem walk [27] and stair-climbing endurance [48]).

The other studies which have shown functional improvements from nonweight-bearing strength training programmes have tended to be on weaker or less active people. The study which has shown the most substantial functional effect of strength training [32] was among frail nursing home residents. Other studies have been among the functionally impaired [36] and older people with osteoarthritis and physical disability [18]. It therefore appears that these people were below threshold levels of strength prior to the intervention.

Functional benefits have been demonstrated when strength training is undertaken in combination with other types of training. One such study of both strength and endurance training [49] was conducted in a nursing home setting, where participants are likely to have also had low initial levels of both strength and endurance. Work by Judge et al. showed that a programme of strength training combined with endurance and balance training improved balance [50] and gait velocity [25] among community dwellers. However, the relative benefits of the different interventions could not be assessed with this study design.

Rooks et al. [51], have tried to apply the principles of strength training to practice of everyday tasks among healthy older people. In addition to seated knee extension exercise, subjects carried out weighted stair-climbing and resisted plantar flexion exercises. This lead to increased strength as well as improved performance on a number of weight-bearing tasks (stair-climbing, single leg balance and ability to reach down to the floor in standing). Interestingly, improved balance and stair-climbing were also noted in a walking-trained group. This suggests that other forms of task-related practice may be as effective as resistance training in improving functional abilities. Similarly, Shaw et al. [52] had subjects carry out weight-bearing exercises with weight vests to provide resistance. This led to significant increases in lower limb strength and subjective reports of enhanced functional abilities among the intervention group.

The data reviewed above suggest that weaker older people can show improved functional abilities following traditional nonweight-bearing strength training programmes. However, older people with greater initial muscle strength do not show such a carry-over. These individuals may have the capacity to improve functional ability with strength training in weight bearing or skill training. Thus, the principles of specificity of training may be most important among stronger older adults. However, older people with less muscle strength may also derive greater benefit from training programmes designed around these principles, than from nonweight-bearing resistance training. This issue requires further investigation.

Endurance training

Background

Endurance training it is not commonly discussed as a falls prevention strategy. However, a loss of aerobic capacity is associated with increased age [15], and difficulty performing activities of daily living and difficulties in walking and transferring (e.g. from bed to chair) have been consistently associated with an increased risk of falling.

Even seemingly simple physical activities such as walking across a room, getting dressed or climbing stairs have energy requirements associated with them. Therefore, a certain level of cardiovascular fitness is required to successfully undertake such activities. In fact, Morey et al. have found that individuals with a peak oxygen uptake of less that 18 ml/kg per minute report significantly more difficulties performing daily tasks [53]. If a person's cardiovascular system is unable to meet the energy requirements of these simple tasks, functional ability and independence will be severely impaired. Such a person is then likely to become increasingly less active. This lack of activity associated with such low levels of functional ability will in turn contribute to greater losses in cardiovascular fitness and also muscle strength.

Other older people may be able to carry out daily activities successfully, yet they may have a reduced physiological reserve and be operating close to their maximum aerobic capacity [24, 54]. When faced with a task with higher demands (e.g. a flight of stairs) they are unable to meet these energy needs and their poor fitness becomes apparent. Reduced reserve may also become apparent if the person suffers an acute illness followed by a further loss of fitness.

It has now been shown that older people can benefit from fitness training [15, 55]. From their review of 22 studies investigating the effects of aerobic training among older adults, Buchner et al. [40] concluded that 3–12 months of exercise improves aerobic capacity by between 5% and 20%. From their meta-analysis of 29 studies of endurance training among older people, Green et al. [56] found an average increase in maximum oxygen consumption of around 23%. These improvements may well be enough to lead to improved functional abilities and therefore decrease the person's risk of falling. Endurance training also has the potential to improve general health among older people [57–59].

Studies have now established the feasibility of endurance training among community-dwelling older people [55, 60, 61], those requiring institutional care [62], and among people with peripheral vascular disease [63–65], stroke [66], coronary artery disease [67], arthritis [18, 68–70], chronic airflow limitation [71] and following lower limb amputation [72]. One study found that 10 years after a randomized controlled trial of an intervention to encourage walking, people in the walking group still reported more frequent walking for exercise [73].

The most recent American College of Sports Medicine position on exercise for older adults [15] recommends that older adults with sufficient strength and balance should undertake an aerobic exercise programme. Such a programme should first target frequency (at least 3 days per week), then duration (at least 20 minutes) and finally appropriate intensity (40–60% of heart rate reserve or 11–13 on the Borg scale of perceived exertion [74]).

The optimal intensity at which older people should undertake endurance training requires further investigation. While moderate- to high-intensity exercise is recommended to increase fitness [15], light- to moderate-intensity physical activity has been associated with a range of other health benefits [58, 59]. There is also some evidence that fitness benefits can also be obtained among older people from lower intensity (30–45% heart rate reserve) endurance training [75].

However, endurance exercise will not be effective in all settings. Daltroy et al. [76] found a 3-month trial of exercise on a stationary bicycle programme did not significantly improve aerobic capacity among people with rheumatoid disease. In a randomized controlled trial of aerobic exercise in cardiac rehabilitation, a supervised programme involving a combination of centre-based and home-based exercise had a greater effect on fitness than an unsupervised home programme [77]. Despite this, King et al. [78] found that home-based endurance exercise was as effective as group-based exercise and 12-month adherence rates were higher in the home-based groups in a randomized controlled trial.

A range of endurance training strategies are available for older people. These include; group exercise classes, walking programmes, treadmill walking or running, stationary cycles and arm cranking. Strategies need to be appropriate for individuals and will depend in part on their level of fitness and skill.

Although in the general aged population the risks associated with inactivity are probably greater than those associated with physical activity [15], endurance training is contraindicated in some individuals. As for strength training, it is important that proper screening takes place before aerobic exercise programmes are undertaken [15, 79–82].

Effects on falls and falls risk

Several randomized trials have evaluated the effects of endurance training on falls and falls risk. One of the studies which found an effect of exercise on falls rates included endurance training [4]. This study found that both endurance training and a combination of strength and endurance training led to increased aerobic capacity, but neither intervention led to improved balance or gait.

Falls risk factors can be modified by endurance training. Rooks et al. [51] found a walking programme conducted in a group setting led to improved tandem and single-leg stance and improved stair-climbing speed. Buchner et al. [83] compared three different endurance training programmes, and found that leg strength was improved by walking, use of a stationary cycle and an 'aerobics' class. Gait speed and self-reported physical ability were also improved in the walking group. In a study of 100 people with rheumatoid arthritis, van den Ende et al. [69] found greater improvements in aerobic capacity, strength and joint mobility with 12 weeks of aerobic (weight-bearing exercise and stationary cycle at 70–85% HRmax) training compared with isometric and range-of-motion exercises (group, individual and home).

Effects on functional abilities

Although endurance training has the potential to lead to improvements in functional abilities, most studies of aerobic training have not measured these abilities. As with muscle strength, it is likely that there is a nonlinear relationship between fitness and functional ability, and that threshold levels of fitness are required for particular tasks. It would be reasonable to expect aerobic training to have a greater effect on the functional abilities of deconditioned people, than on those who had sufficient aerobic fitness to complete the task in question, prior to the intervention.

In one of the few studies designed to address this question, Ettinger et al. [18] compared both aerobic (group exercise 50–70% of HRR) and resistance training (10RM) with health education, among 439 older people with osteoarthritic knees causing pain and disability. The participants attended 3 months of group exercise then completed a 15-month home programme. When compared with health education, both aerobic and resistance training led to decreased pain and disability, and improved 6-minute walk distance, stair-climbing ability, performance of a lift-and-carry task, and the time taken to get out of a car. Only aerobic training led to an increased aerobic capacity, and neither intervention increased strength.

Individual physiotherapy intervention

Background

Everyday tasks (such as standing up from a seated position, remaining balanced while standing and walking) can be considered to be motor skills. Among older people, performance of these tasks may be hampered by a range of physical impairments. As well as increasing the risk of falling, this suboptimal motor performance may reduce a person's independence and thus quality of life. As with any other skill, performance of functional tasks may be improved with motor training and practice.

In recent years, many physiotherapists have adopted a motor learning model of rehabilitation [84, 85] in which the client becomes the learner and the therapist the movement coach. This differs from more traditional models in which the patient is the passive recipient of a therapy [86]. In this model, practice, feedback and the environmental context are seen as crucial to the acquisition of motor skills. To properly assess the effects of the intervention, objective measures of motor performance (e.g. lowest height chair from which a person can stand up, time to walk 10 m) must be used. When faced with an older person with impaired motor skills, the role of the physiotherapist is to assess motor performance, analyse the cause of any movement problems, develop an intervention programme tailored to these problems, and assess the effects of this intervention programme [84, 85].

Potential causes for observed gait problems among people following stroke are well summarized by a group of Sydney physiotherapists [87, 88]. These have been divided into stance and swing phase problems and describe the inability to generate sufficient muscle force or the production of excessive muscle force at particular points of the gait cycle, and tissue changes preventing normal joint angle at particular points in the gait cycle. For example, increased knee flexion in stance phase could be caused by an inability to produce sufficient active tension with the knee extensor muscles, production of excessive active tension with the knee flexor muscles, or shortening of the knee flexor muscles or decreases in compliance of other tissues on the flexor aspect of the knee. Similar causes may impair walking among the general frail aged population.

Practice is a vital component of motor learning. A relationship between the amount of practice undertaken and the outcome achieved has been demonstrated in several noncontrolled studies of people following stroke [89, 90]. As the type of practice done is probably important to skill learning, practice should be relevant to the particular task being trained [85]. The learner's ongoing motivation is likely to affect the amount of practice done and they are likely to carry out a greater volume of practice if this is seen as relevant to the goal (e.g. better ability to balance in standing) [91].

In order to identify and address particular motor problems, older people at high risk of falling may benefit from this individualized approach rather than a more general exercise programme. In addition, physiotherapists have an important role to play in teaching older people to get up from the floor after having fallen [92], and in prescribing the other types of exercise described in this chapter.

Effects on falls and falls risk

Research is yet to look at the effect of individual (one-on-one) training on falls. However, studies have shown improvements in a number of functional abilities which have also been identified as falls risk factors.

Effects on functional abilities

Randomized trials have evaluated various types of individualized motor training. Among people following stroke, Dean and Shepherd [93] showed an improvement in lower limb force generation and standing-up ability following motor training and supervised practice of reaching in sitting. Richards et al. [94] showed increased gait velocity with intensive task-specific training when compared with other approaches to stroke rehabilitation. In general, randomized controlled trials have found additional benefits from more intensive physiotherapy and/or occupational therapy intervention among people following stroke [95, 96].

Two studies have looked at individual balance training. Wolfson et al. [31] reported that balance training (involving various conditions with a computerized platform with feedback, in standing, while sitting on a balance ball and while walking on foam and on a narrow beam) led to improved balance (as measured by the sensory organization test, single stance time, and voluntary limits of stability). This study also involved strength training, which did not have such a positive effect on measures of balance. Hu and Woollacott [97, 98] conducted a randomized controlled trial among 26 active people aged 65–90. Intervention subjects practised standing with eyes open or closed, head neutral or extended, and on a firm or foam support surface. This training had the effect of improving stability in five of the eight training conditions, with some differences between the groups persisting 4 weeks after the intervention.

In an 8-month randomized trial of physiotherapy intervention (which included balance and coordination training as well as more general exercise) among 194 frail nursing home residents, Mulrow et al. [99] found no change in balance performance (Physical Disability Index subscale) but an increase in independent mobility among the intervention group.

Other noncontrolled studies have also found benefits of individual training targeting impairments identified on assessment of the person's physical abilities. Such benefits have been found among older people following hip fracture [100] and among younger people following traumatic brain injury [101]. Another noncontrolled study suggests that a greater volume of physical therapy input is associated with enhanced functional outcomes among people with acute orthopaedic problems [102].

Several of the studies have found improved functional abilities following this approach. Future research could compare the effect of individual motor training on functional abilities with the effects of other strategies, such as strength training.

General exercise

Background

This section examines other exercise programmes which aim to reduce falls risk and improve motor function among older people yet do not comply with the prescription principles outlined above for strength or endurance training. These strategies are discussed in terms of group exercise and unsupervised home exercise.

Effects on falls and falls risk: group exercise

Our group has designed a group exercise programme which is effective in improving performance on a number of measures of fall risk [103–105]. In a 12-month randomized controlled trial of this exercise programme in 197 women, improvements were evident in lower limb strength (ankle dorsiflexion, knee flexion and extension, and hip flexion and extension), reaction time, neuromuscular control, postural sway, maximal balance range and coordinated stability in the exercise group. The exercise subjects also showed significantly increased walking speed, cadence, stride length and decreased stride times. The intervention involved twice-weekly one-hour group exercise classes. These included warm-up, conditioning (aerobic exercises, strengthening exercises and activities for balance, flexibility, endurance and coordination), stretching and relaxation components.

As discussed previously, Tai Chi conducted in a group setting has been shown to reduce the risk of multiple falls by 48% [106]. A number of other randomized controlled trials have investigated group exercise programmes among relatively healthy older people. Programmes which have been found to be effective in fall risk factor modification generally involve exercise carried out in weight-bearing positions which involve controlled body movements (i.e. weight transference). Improvements among exercise subjects have been shown in: strength [83, 107–109], balance [83, 110], gait velocity [110], range of movement [108, 111], life satisfaction [108], maximum physical exertion level [108], and perceived health status [108, 109]. Bravo et al. [109] report that their 12-month programme of weight-bearing exercises, aerobic dancing and flexibility exercises had the additional benefit of stabilizing spinal bone mineral density (which deteriorated in the control group) but did not affect femoral neck bone mineral density.

However, not all group exercise programmes improve all measures of fall risk. For example, it has been found that seated flexibility exercises had no effect on strength and gait velocity [25], and that there was no additional strength benefit from exercise with light weights than unweighted exercise [107], a 20-minute programme of stretching and nonresisted strengthening exercise did not affect strength or postural sway [111], and a Tai Chi programme did not lead to improved leg muscle strength [3].

The effects of group exercise have also been investigated with randomized controlled trials among frailer people living in supported accommodation. McMurdo et al. [112, 113] compared the effects of a seated exercise class (involving isometric gravity-resisted exercises) with those of a reminiscence group and found increased quadriceps strength, spinal flexion range of motion, and impaired activities of daily living ability among the exercise group. Self-rating of depression decreased in both groups but this decrease was significantly greater among the exercise group. No change in postural sway or reaction time was evident. Although this intervention was of a relatively low intensity and conducted in a seated position it appears to have been intense enough to improve functional performance among this group.

In contrast, other programmes have failed to find beneficial effects of group exercise among frailer populations [114]. In fact, Crilly et al. [115] found no improvement in balance abilities among both intervention and control groups after a 12-week group exercise programme.

From the studies summarized above, it seems important that the interventions involved in a group exercise programme are of sufficient intensity. It also seems that exercise can improve balance abilities if it involves practice of movement in standing. It may be that practice controlling large movements of the centre of mass is the most effective way to enhance balance. It is interesting that some group exercise programmes can lead to an increase in muscle strength without consciously applying the principles of high-resistance training. Although these increases in strength tend to be smaller in magnitude than those gained in resistance training programmes, they may still be sufficient to reduce falls risk.

Effects on falls and falls risk: home exercise

The study by Campbell et al. [6], discussed previously, demonstrated that home exercise programmes have the potential to decrease fall rates. This programme involved a combination of weight-bearing and nonweight-bearing exercises resisted with light weights. While this study also found improvements in balance and ability to stand up from sitting, no change was evident in gait or stair-climbing speed, functional reach or strength.

We found improved strength and walking speed, but no change in functional reach or postural sway, following a 1-month home exercise programme for people following hip fracture [116]. This programme involved the lateral step-up or 'weight-bearing' exercise as described for use among people following stroke [89]. The participant stands with one foot resting on a block and the other beside the block. The leg on the block is then straightened so that the other leg lifts off the ground and the body-weight is supported on one leg. Hand support is used if necessary. Thus the person practises using the leg extensor muscles to support the body against gravity, as is required in the stance phase of walking [117].

Several other randomized controlled trials have found improvements in falls risk factors with home exercise programmes. Jette et al. [118] trialled a 6-month programme of exercise resisted with elastic sheeting among 215 older people with disability. They also used a motivational video and a range of behavioural strategies which included rewards for mailing completed exercise logs. This programme led to improved strength and balance, and decreased disability but did not affect gait. In an earlier study [119], a similar programme over 12–15 weeks among 102 non-disabled community-dwellers led to improved strength among the younger subjects and psychological benefits among male subjects.

Following a randomized trial of 6 months of daily lower limb exercise, O'Reilly et al. [120] report decreased pain and improved function among the exercise group. This intervention involved isometric quadriceps exercise in sitting, isotonic quadriceps exercise in sitting, isotonic hamstrings exercise in lying, quadriceps exercise with resistance band in sitting, and stepping up and down one step. In a non-randomized controlled trial, Sashika et al. [121] found improved gait speed and cadence with home-based non-resisted strength training and balance exercise, among people following hip replacement.

As several studies have failed to show significant improvements in any outcome variables with home exercise programmes [122, 123], it seems that the type of intervention is also important for home exercise programmes: a home exercise programme will not necessarily lead to improvements in strength or balance.

Effects on functional abilities

As outlined above, group exercise programmes conducted primarily in weight-bearing positions have been shown to lead to improved functional abilities for people with a range of initial abilities. Such weight-bearing exercise is clearly of relevance to everyday tasks such as standing and walking. Similarly, several of the studies outlined above demonstrate that home exercise has the potential to improve functional abilities. As with other forms of exercise, the extent of functional improvement will probably depend on the exact nature of the programme.

Setting

The different types of exercise described above can be conducted in various settings. The most preferable setting for an individual will depend on lifestyle, other responsibilities and the person's ability to maintain motivation. Exercise can be conducted in a group or individually, can have various levels of supervision, and can be conducted within a healthcare centre, in a community setting or within the person's home.

Advantages of exercise within a group setting include support and assistance from an instructor, the structure provided by having a regular period of time allocated to exercise, the mutual encouragement and socialization provided by a group, and the enjoyable use of music. General exercise is often carried out in a group setting and resistance training has also been shown to be effective in this setting [4, 25]. However, some individuals may not enjoy group environments and may prefer to exercise alone or with one other person. For some older people it may be difficult to physically access venues where exercise classes are held (e.g. due to frailty and/or dependence on others for transport), or to find time to attend a regular class (e.g. due to responsibilities of caring for a partner or grandchildren, or social engagements). There is evidence that strength training can be successfully undertaken at home either alone [47] or supervised [36]. Endurance training can be as effective at home as in a group setting [78], In fact, in their randomized controlled trial [78], King et al. found that 12-month adherence rates were higher in home-based groups. It has been argued that supervised home exercise programmes are the ideal way of promoting physical activity [124] as they are cheaper to establish than group exercise, cater for those who dislike group exercise, yet minimize the risks associated with unsupervised home exercise among frailer people.

Equipment needs may also limit venues where exercise can be undertaken. Resistance training often involves expensive nonportable equipment used under supervision in a health care facility. However, after full assessment, community-dwelling older people could be taught to use exercise machines in a local gymnasium. In addition, several authors have shown increased strength among older people with the application of the principles of resistance training to more readily available tools such as free weights, body weight and elastic sheeting [36, 47, 51].

Different types of exercise intervention require differing levels of supervision. For example, motor training requires ongoing input from a physiotherapist in training sessions at a healthcare facility or within the person's home [93]. However, the ongoing practice/exercise undertaken by the client after input from the physiotherapist is also crucial. Exercise diaries or practice records may assist in this. A set of exercise cards for task-related practice has been developed by the Physiotherapy Department at St Joseph's Hospital in Sydney. Examples of these are shown in Figure 8.1.

There is evidence that ongoing supervision and support is important in maintaining adherence to exercise [76, 77, 125] and the efficacy of this exercise. Kerschan et al. found that while 5–10 year compliance with an unvarying home exercise programme was reasonable (36%), the resulting intensity was not enough to reduce fracture risk [126]. Although ongoing supervision of exercise programmes may appear expensive, this may be outweighed by the potential savings from falls prevented by a successful programme.

The ideal exercise setting therefore depends on the nature of the exercise, the

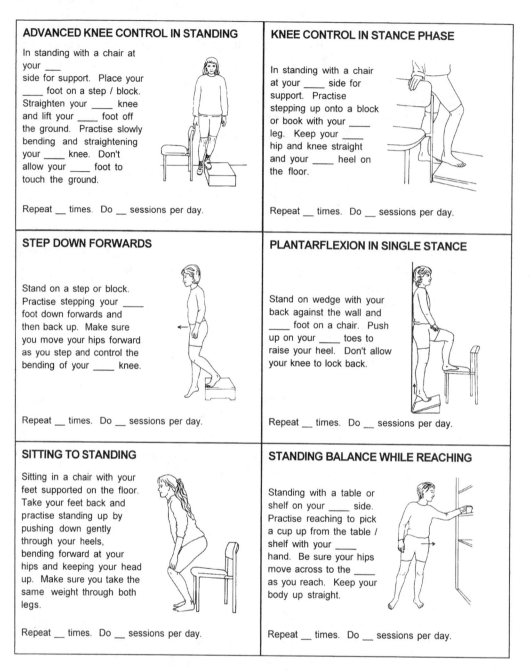

ADVANCED KNEE CONTROL IN STANDING

In standing with a chair at your ____
side for support. Place your ____ foot on a step / block. Straighten your ____ knee and lift your ____ foot off the ground. Practise slowly bending and straightening your ____ knee. Don't allow your ____ foot to touch the ground.

Repeat __ times. Do __ sessions per day.

KNEE CONTROL IN STANCE PHASE

In standing with a chair at your ____ side for support. Practise stepping up onto a block or book with your ____ leg. Keep your ____ hip and knee straight and your ____ heel on the floor.

Repeat __ times. Do __ sessions per day.

STEP DOWN FORWARDS

Stand on a step or block. Practise stepping your ____ foot down forwards and then back up. Make sure you move your hips forward as you step and control the bending of your ____ knee.

Repeat __ times. Do __ sessions per day.

PLANTARFLEXION IN SINGLE STANCE

Stand on wedge with your back against the wall and ____ foot on a chair. Push up on your ____ toes to raise your heel. Don't allow your knee to lock back.

Repeat __ times. Do __ sessions per day.

SITTING TO STANDING

Sitting in a chair with your feet supported on the floor. Take your feet back and practise standing up by pushing down gently through your heels, bending forward at your hips and keeping your head up. Make sure you take the same weight through both legs.

Repeat __ times. Do __ sessions per day.

STANDING BALANCE WHILE REACHING

Standing with a table or shelf on your ____ side. Practise reaching to pick a cup up from the table / shelf with your ____ hand. Be sure your hips move across to the ____ as you reach. Keep your body up straight.

Repeat __ times. Do __ sessions per day.

Fig. 8.1.   Examples of exercise cards. Reproduced with permission from St Joseph's Hospital Physiotherapy Department, Sydney, Australia.

purpose of this exercise (i.e. whether it aims to address particular deficits), and the personality and social situation of the older person.

Conclusion

While adequate attention must be given to safety issues [20], there is certainly much scope to increase levels of exercise participation among older people. As well as assisting in the prevention of falls, this will provide a range of additional health benefits [59, 124]. Indeed, there is now mounting evidence that several different exercise intervention strategies can reduce fall rates among older people. Successful strategies used in studies have included balance training, Tai Chi, strength and/or endurance group exercise and a home exercise programme.

There is certainly strong evidence that exercise can improve performance on key physical falls risk factors. Exercise which is more intensive and/or carried out in a weight-bearing position has been found to be most effective.

As it is not the case that each form of exercise will reduce the risk of falling for every older person, careful consideration should be given to the type of exercise prescribed. As with other falls prevention interventions, exercise will be more effective if targeted to the person's particular deficits and lifestyle.

REFERENCES

1 Hadley E. The science of the art of geriatric medicine. *Journal of the American Medical Association* 1995;273:1381–3.

2 Province MA, Hadley EC, Hornbrook MC, et al. The effects of exercise on falls in elderly patients. A preplanned meta-analysis of the FICSIT Trials. Frailty and Injuries: Cooperative Studies of Intervention Techniques. *Journal of the American Medical Association* 1995;273:1341–7.

3 Wolf SL, Barnhart HX, Kutner NG, McNeely E, Coogler C, Xu T. Reducing frailty and falls in older persons: an investigation of Tai Chi and computerized balance training. *Journal of the American Geriatrics Society* 1996;44:489–97.

4 Buchner DM, Cress ME, de Lateur BJ, et al. The effect of strength and endurance training on gait, balance, fall risk, and health services use in community-living older adults. *Journals of Gerontology. Series A, Biological Sciences and Medical Sciences* 1997;52:M218–24.

5 Tinetti ME, Baker DI, McAvay G, et al. A multifactorial intervention to reduce the risk of falling among elderly people living in the community. *New England Journal of Medicine* 1994;331:821–7.

6 Campbell AJ, Robertson MC, Gardner MM, Norton RN, Tilyard MW, Buchner DM. randomized controlled trial of a general practice programme of home based exercise to prevent falls in elderly women. *British Medical Journal* 1997;315:1065–9.

7   Gillespie LD, Gillespie WJ, Cumming R, Lamb SE, Rowe BH. Interventions for preventing falls in the elderly (Cochrane Review). The Cochrane Library, issue 3. Oxford: Update Software, 1999.

8   Jones D, Rutherford O, Parker D. Physiological changes in skeletal muscle as a result of strength training. *Quarterly Journal of Experimental Physiology* 1989;74:233–256.

9   DeLorme T, Watkins A: *Progressive resistance exercise: technical and medical application*. New York: Appleton-Century-Crofts, 1951.

10 Fleck S, Kraemer W. *Designing resistance training programs*, 2nd ed. Champaign, IL: Human Kinetics, 1997.

11 Nelson M, Wernick S. *Strong women stay young*. Port Melbourne: Lothian Books, 1997.

12 Westcott W, Baechle T. *Strength training past 50: for fitness and performance through the years*. Champaign, IL: Human Kinetics, 1998.

13 ACSM. American College of Sports Medicine position stand. The recommended quantity and quality of exercise for developing and maintaining cardiorespiratory and muscular fitness, and flexibility in healthy adults. *Medicine and Science in Sports and Exercise* 1998;30:975–91.

14 Feigenbaum M, Pollock M. Strength training: rationale for current guidelines for adult fitness programmes. *The Physician and Sportsmedicine* 1997;25:44–64.

15 ACSM. American College of Sports Medicine position stand. Exercise and physical activity for older adults. *Medicine and Science in Sports and Exercise* 1998;30:992–1008.

16 Hunter GR, Treuth MS. Relative training intensity and increases in strength in older women. *Journal of Strength and Conditioning Research* 1995;9:188–91.

17 Taaffe DR, Pruitt L, Pyka G, Guido D, Marcus R. Comparative effects of high- and low-intensity resistance training on thigh muscle strength, fiber area, and tissue composition in elderly women. *Clinical Physiology* 1996;16:381–92.

18 Ettinger WH Jr, Burns R, Messier SP, et al. A randomized trial comparing aerobic exercise and resistance exercise with a health education programme in older adults with knee osteoarthritis. The fitness arthritis and seniors trial (FAST). *Journal of the American Medical Association* 1997;277:25–31.

19 Ghilarducci LE, Holly R, Amsterdam E. Effects of high resistance training in coronary artery disease. *American Journal of Cardiology* 1989;64:866–70.

20 ACSM. American College of Sports Medicine and American Heart Association joint position statement. Recommendations for cardiovascular screening, staffing, and emergency policies at health/fitness facilities. *Medicine and Science in Sports and Exercise* 1998;30:1009–18.

21 Hurley BF. Age, gender, and muscular strength. *Journals of Gerontology. Series A, Biological Sciences and Medical Sciences* 1995;50:41–4.

22 Campbell AJ, Borrie MJ, Spears GF. Risk factors for falls in a community-based prospective study of people 70 years and older. *Journal of Gerontology* 1989;44:M112–17.

23 Lord SR, Ward JA, Williams P, Anstey KJ. Physiological factors associated with falls in older community-dwelling women. *Journal of the American Geriatrics Society* 1994;42:1110–17.

24 Buchner DM, Wagner EH. Preventing frail health. *Clinics in Geriatric Medicine* 1992;8:1–17.

25 Judge JO, Underwood M, Gennosa T. Exercise to improve gait velocity in older persons. *Archives of Physical Medicine and Rehabilitation* 1993;74:400–6.

26 Nichols JF, Omizo DK, Peterson KK, Nelson KP. Efficacy of heavy-resistance training for active women over sixty: muscular strength, body composition, and programme adherence. *Journal of the American Geriatrics Society* 1993;41:205–10.

27 Nelson ME, Fiatarone MA, Morganti CM, Trice I, Greenberg RA, Evans WJ. Effects of high-intensity strength training on multiple risk factors for osteoporotic fractures: a randomized controlled trial. *Journal of the American Medical Association* 1994;272:1909–14.

28 Pyka G, Lindenberger E, Charette S, Marcus R. Muscle strength and fiber adaptations to a year-long resistance training programme in elderly men and women. *Journal of Gerontology* 1994;49:M22–7.

29 McCartney N, Hicks AL, Martin J, Webber CE. Long-term resistance training in the elderly: effects on dynamic strength, exercise capacity, muscle, and bone. *Journals of Gerontology. Series A, Biological Sciences and Medical Sciences* 1995;50:B97–104.

30 Morganti C, Nelson M, Fiatarone M, et al. Strength improvements with 1 year of progressive resistance training in older women. *Medicine and Science in Sports and Exercise* 1995;27:906–12.

31 Wolfson L, Whipple R, Derby C, et al. Balance and strength training in older adults: intervention gains and Tai Chi maintenance. *Journal of the American Geriatrics Society* 1996;44:498–506.

32 Fiatarone MA, O'Neill EF, Ryan ND, et al. Exercise training and nutritional supplementation for physical frailty in very elderly people. *New England Journal of Medicine* 1994;330:1769–75.

33 Fiatarone MA, Marks EC, Ryan ND, Meredith CN, Lipsitz LA, Evans WJ. High-intensity strength training in nonagenarians. Effects on skeletal muscle. *Journal of the American Medical Association* 1990;263:3029–34.

34 Fisher NM, Pendergast DR, Calkins E. Muscle rehabilitation in impaired elderly nursing home residents. *Archives of Physical Medicine & Rehabilitation* 1991;72:181–5.

35 Buchner DM, Larson EB, Wagner EH, Koepsell TD, de Lateur BJ. Evidence for a non-linear relationship between leg strength and gait speed. *Age and Ageing* 1996;25:386–91.

36 Chandler JM, Duncan PW, Kochersberger G, Studenski S. Is lower extremity strength gain associated with improvement in physical performance and disability in frail, community-dwelling elders? *Archives of Physical Medicine and Rehabilitation* 1998;79:24–30.

37 Skelton D, Young A. Are the National Fitness Survey strength and power thresholds for performance of everyday tasks too high? *Journal of Physiology* 1993;473:84P.

38 Brown M, Sinacore DR, Host HH. The relationship of strength to function in the older adult. *Journals of Gerontology. Series A, Biological Sciences and Medical Sciences* 1995;50:55–9.

39 Rantanen T, Era P, Heikkinen E. Maximal isometric knee extension strength and stair-mounting ability in 75- and 80-year-old men and women. *Scandinavian Journal of Rehabilitation Medicine* 1996;28:89–93.

40 Buchner DM, Beresford SA, Larson EB, LaCroix AZ, Wagner EH. Effects of physical activity on health status in older adults. II. Intervention studies. *Annual Review of Public Health* 1992;13:469–88.

41 Sale D, MacDougall D. Specificity in strength training: a review for the coach and athlete. *Canadian Journal of Applied Sports Sciences* 1981;6:87–92.

42 Wilson G, Murphy A, Walshe A. The specificity of strength training: the effect of posture. *European Journal of Applied Physiology* 1996;73:346–52.

43 Kanehisa H, Miyashita M. Specificity of velocity in strength training. *European Journal of Applied Physiology* 1983;52:104–6.

44 Lindh M. Increase of muscle strength from isometric quadriceps exercises at different knee angles. *Scandanavian Journal of Rehabilitation Medicine* 1979;11:33–6.

45 Rutherford O. Muscular coordination and strength training. Implications for injury rehabilitation. *Sports Medicine* 1988;5:196–202.

46 Judge JO, Whipple RH, Wolfson LI. Effects of resistive and balance exercises on isokinetic strength in older persons. *Journal of the American Geriatrics Society* 1994;42:937–46.

47 Skelton DA, Young A, Greig CA, Malbut KE. Effects of resistance training on strength, power, and selected functional abilities of women aged 75 and older. *Journal of the American Geriatrics Society* 1995;43:1081–7.

48 McCartney N, Hicks AL, Martin J, Webber CE. A longitudinal trial of weight training in the elderly: continued improvements in year 2. *Journals of Gerontology. Series A, Biological Sciences and Medical Sciences* 1996;51:B425–33.

49 Sauvage LR Jr, Myklebust BM, Crow-Pan J, et al. A clinical trial of strengthening and aerobic exercise to improve gait and balance in elderly male nursing home residents. *American Journal of Physical Medicine & Rehabilitation* 1992;71:333–42.

50 Judge JO, Lindsey C, Underwood M, Winsemius D. Balance improvements in older women: effects of exercise training. *Physical Therapy* 1993;73:254–65.

51 Rooks DS, Kiel DP, Parsons C, Hayes WC. Self-paced resistance training and walking exercise in community-dwelling older adults: effects on neuromotor performance. *Journals of Gerontology. Series A, Biological Sciences and Medical Sciences* 1997;52:M161–8.

52 Shaw JM, Snow CM. Weighted vest exercise improves indices of fall risk in older women. *Journals of Gerontology. Series A, Biological Sciences and Medical Sciences* 1998;53:M53–8.

53 Morey M, Pieper C, Cornoni-Huntley J. Is there a threshold between peak oxygen uptake and self-reported physical functioning in older adults. *Medicine and Science in Sports and Exercise* 1998;30:1223–9.

54 Buchner DM, Cress ME, Wagner EH, de Lateur BJ. The role of exercise in fall prevention: developing targeting criteria for exercise programmes. In: Vellas B, Toupet M, Rubenstein L, Albarede JL, Christen Y, editors. *Falls, balance and gait disorders in the elderly.* Paris: Elsevier, 1992.

55 Posner JD, Gorman KM, Windsor-Landsberg L, et al. Low to moderate intensity endurance training in healthy older adults: physiological responses after four months. *Journal of the American Geriatrics Society* 1992;40:1–7.

56 Green JS, Crouse SF. The effects of endurance training on functional capacity in the elderly: a meta-analysis. *Medicine and Science in Sports and Exercise* 1995;27:920–6.

57 Posner JD, Gorman KM, Gitlin LN, et al. Effects of exercise training in the elderly on the occurrence and time to onset of cardiovascular diagnoses. *Journal of the American Geriatrics Society* 1990;38:205–10.

58 Haskell W. Health consequences of physical activity: understanding and challenges regarding dose–response. *Medicine and Science in Sports and Exercise* 1994;26:649–660.

59 Pate RR, Pratt M, Blair SN, et al. Physical activity and public health. A recommendation from the Centers for Disease Control and Prevention and the American College of Sports Medicine. *Journal of the American Medical Association* 1995;273:402–7.

60 Stevenson JS, Topp R. Effects of moderate and low intensity long-term exercise by older adults. *Research in Nursing and Health* 1990;13:209–18.

61 Morey MC, Cowper PA, Feussner JR, DiPasquale RC, Crowley GM, Sullivan RJ Jr. Two-year trends in physical performance following supervised exercise among community-dwelling older veterans. *Journal of the American Geriatrics Society* 1991;39:549–54.

62 Naso F, Carner E, Blankfort-Doyle W, Coughey K. Endurance training in the elderly nursing home patient. *Archives of Physical Medicine and Rehabilitation* 1990;71:241–3.

63 Hiatt WR, Wolfel EE, Meier RH, Regensteiner JG. Superiority of treadmill walking exercise versus strength training for patients with peripheral arterial disease. Implications for the mechanism of the training response. *Circulation* 1994;90:1866–74.

64 Leng GC, Fowler B, Ernst E. Exercise for intermittent claudication (Cochrane Review). In: The Cochrane Library, issue 3. Oxford: Update Software, 1999.

65 Brandsma J, Robeer B, van den Heuvel S, Smith B, Wittens C, Oostendorp R. The effect of exercises on walking distance of patients with intermittent claudication: a study of randomized controlled trials. *Physical Therapy* 1998;78:278–88.

66 Potempa K, Lopez M, Braun L, Szidon J, Fogg L, Tincknell T. Physiological outcomes of aerobic exercise training in hemiparetic stroke patients. *Stroke* 1995;26:101–5.

67 Fletcher B, Dunbar S, Felner J, et al. Exercise testing and training in physically disabled men with clinical evidence of coronary artery disease. *American Journal of Cardiology* 1994;73:170–4.

68 Minor MA, Hewett JE, Webel RR, Anderson SK, Kay DR. Efficacy of physical conditioning exercise in patients with rheumatoid arthritis and osteoarthritis. *Arthritis and Rheumatism* 1989;32:1396–405.

69 van den Ende CH, Hazes JM, le Cessie S, et al. Comparison of high- and low-intensity training in well-controlled rheumatoid arthritis. Results of a randomized clinical trial. *Annals of the Rheumatic Diseases* 1996;55:798–805.

70 van den Ende C, Vliet Vlieland T, Munneke M, Hazes J. Dynamic exercise therapy in rheumatoid arthritis: a systematic review. *British Journal of Rheumatology* 1998;37:677–87.

71 Nosworthy J, Barter C, Thomas S, Flynn M. An evaluation of three elements of pulmonary rehabilitation. *Australian Journal of Physiotherapy* 1992;38:189–93.

72 Pitetti K, Snell P, Stray-Gundersen J, Gottschalk F. Aerobic training exercises for individuals who had amputation of the lower limb. *The Journal of Bone and Joint Surgery (Am)* 1987;69:914–21.

73 Pereira MA, Kriska AM, Day RD, Cauley JA, LaPorte RE, Kuller LH. A randomized walking trial in postmenopausal women: effects on physical activity and health 10 years later. *Archives of Internal Medicine* 1998;158:1695–701.

74 Borg G. Psychophysical basis of perceived exertion. *Medicine and Science in Sports and Exercise* 1982;14:377–381.

75 Badenhop DT, Cleary PA, Schaal SF, Fox EL, Bartels RL. Physiological adjustments to higher- or lower-intensity exercise in elders. *Medicine and Science in Sports and Exercise* 1983;15:496–502.

76 Daltroy L, Robb-Nicholson C, Iversen M, Wright E, Liang M. Effectiveness of minimally supervised home aerobic training in patients with systemic rheumatic disease. *British Journal of Rheumatology* 1995;34:1064–9.

77 Kugler J, Dimsdale JE, Hartley LH, Sherwood J. Hospital supervised vs home exercise in cardiac rehabilitation: effects on aerobic fitness, anxiety, and depression. *Archives of Physical Medicine and Rehabilitation* 1990;71:322–5.

78 King AC, Haskell WL, Taylor CB, Kraemer HC, DeBusk RF. Group- vs home-based exercise training in healthy older men and women. A community-based clinical trial. *Journal of the American Medical Association* 1991;266:1535–42.

79 Pollock M, Wilmore J. *Exercise in health and disease: evaluation and prescription for prevention and rehabilitation.* Philadelphia: Saunders, 1990.

80 ACSM. American College of Sports Medicine. *Guidelines for exercise testing and prescription,* 4th ed. Philadelphia: Lea and Febiger, 1991.

81 Fletcher G, Balady G, Froelicher V, Hartley L, Haskell W, Pollock M. Exercise standards: a statement for healthcare professionals from the American Heart Association. *Circulation* 1995;91:580–615.

82 ACSM American Colleage of Sports Medicine. *Resource manual for guidelines for exercise testing and prescription,* 3rd ed. Baltimore: Williams and Wilkins, 1998.

83 Buchner DM, Cress ME, de Lateur BJ, et al. A comparison of the effects of three types of endurance training on balance and other fall risk factors in older adults. *Aging* 1997;9:112–19.

84 Carr J, Shepherd R. A motor learning model for stroke rehabilitation. *Physiotherapy* 1989;75:372–80.

85 Carr J, Shepherd R. *Neurological rehabilitation: optimizing motor performance.* Oxford: Butterworth-Heinemann, 1998.

86 Gordon J. Assumptions underlying physical therapy intervention: theoretical and historical perspectives. In: Carr J, Shepherd R, Gordon J, et al., editors. *Movement science: foundations for physical therapy in rehabilitation.* Maryland: Aspen, 1987.

87 Moseley A, Wales A, Herbert R, Schurr K, Moore S. Observation and analysis of hemiplegic gait: stance phase. *Australian Journal of Physiotherapy* 1993;39:259–67.

88 Moore S, Schurr K, Wales A, Moseley A, Herbert R. Observation and analysis of hemiplegic gait: swing phase. *Australian Journal of Physiotherapy* 1993;39:271–8.

89 Nugent JA, Schurr KA, Adams RD. A dose–response relationship between amount of weight-bearing exercise and walking outcome following cerebrovascular accident. *Archives of Physical Medicine and Rehabilitation* 1994;75:399–402.

90 Butefisch C, Hummelsheim H, Denzler P, Mauritz K-H. Repetitive training of isolated movements improves the outcome of motor rehabilitation of the centrally paretic hand. *Journal of the Neurological Sciences* 1995;130:59–68.

91 Hsieh CL, Nelson DL, Smith DA, Peterson CQ. A comparison of performance in added-

purpose occupations and rote exercise for dynamic standing balance in persons with hemiplegia. *American Journal of Occupational Therapy* 1996;50:10–6.

92 Reece AC, Simpson JM. Preparing older people to cope after a fall. *Physiotherapy* 1996;82:227–35.

93 Dean CM, Shepherd RB. Task-related training improves performance of seated reaching tasks after stroke: a randomized controlled trial. *Stroke* 1997;28:722–8.

94 Richards CL, Malouin F, Wood-Dauphinee S, Williams JI, Bouchard JP, Brunet D. Task-specific physical therapy for optimization of gait recovery in acute stroke patients. *Archives of Physical Medicine and Rehabilitation* 1993;74:612–20.

95 Kwakkel G, Wagenaar R, Koelman T, Lankhorst G, Koetsier J. Effects of intensity of rehabilitation after stroke: a research synthesis. *Stroke* 1997;28:1550–6.

96 Langhorne P, Wagenaar R, Partridge C. Physiotherapy after stroke: more is better? *Physiotherapy Research International* 1996;1:75–88.

97 Hu MH, Woollacott MH. Multisensory training of standing balance in older adults, I. Postural stability and one-leg stance balance. *Journal of Gerontology* 1994;49:M52–61.

98 Hu MH, Woollacott MH. Multisensory training of standing balance in older adults, II. Kinematic and electromyographic postural responses. *Journal of Gerontology* 1994;49:M62–71.

99 Mulrow C, Gerety M, Kanten D, et al. A randomized trial of physical rehabilitation for very frail nursing home residents. *Journal of the American Medical Association* 1994;271:519–24.

100 Tinetti ME, Baker DI, Gottschalk M, et al. Systematic home-based physical and functional therapy for older persons after hip fracture. *Archives of Physical Medicine and Rehabilitation* 1997;78:1237–47.

101 Wade L, Canning C, Fowler V, Felmingham K, Baguley I. Changes in postural sway and performance of functional tasks during rehabilitation after traumatic brain injury. *Archives of Physical Medicine and Rehabilitation* 1997;78:1107–11.

102 Roach K, Ally D, Finnerty B, et al. The relationship between duration of physical therapy services in the acute care setting and change in functional status in patients with lower-extremity orthopedic problems. *Physical Therapy* 1998;78:19–24.

103 Lord SR, Ward JA, Williams P, Strudwick M. The effect of a 12-month exercise trial on balance, strength, and falls in older women: a randomized controlled trial. *Journal of the American Geriatrics Society* 1995;43:1198–206.

104 Lord SR, Lloyd DG, Nirui M, Raymond J, Williams P, Stewart RA. The effect of exercise on gait patterns in older women: a randomized controlled trial. *Journals of Gerontology. Series A, Biological Sciences and Medical Sciences* 1996;51:M64–70.

105 Lord SR, Ward JA, Williams P. Exercise effect on dynamic stability in older women: a randomized controlled trial. *Archives of Physical Medicine and Rehabilitation* 1996;77:232–6.

106 Wolf SL, Barnhart HX, Kutner NG, McNeely E, Coogler C, Xu T. Reducing frailty and falls in older persons: an investigation of Tai Chi and computerized balance training. Atlanta FICSIT Group. Frailty and injuries: cooperative studies of intervention techniques. *Journal of the American Geriatrics Society* 1996;44:489–97.

107 Agre JC, Pierce LE, Raab DM, McAdams M, Smith EL. Light resistance and stretching

exercise in elderly women: effect upon strength. *Archives of Physical Medicine and Rehabilitation* 1988;69:273–6.

108 McMurdo ME, Burnett L. Randomized controlled trial of exercise in the elderly. *Gerontology* 1992;38:292–8.

109 Bravo G, Gauthier P, Roy PM, et al. Impact of a 12-month exercise programme on the physical and psychological health of osteopenic women. *Journal of the American Geriatrics Society* 1996;44:756–62.

110 Johansson G, Jarnlo GB. Balance training in 70-year-old women. *Physiotherapy Theory and Practice* 1991;7:121–5.

111 Mills EM. The effect of low-intensity aerobic exercise on muscle strength, flexibility, and balance among sedentary elderly persons. *Nursing Research* 1994;43:207–11.

112 McMurdo ME, Rennie L. A controlled trial of exercise by residents of old people's homes. *Age and Ageing* 1993;22:11–15.

113 McMurdo ME, Rennie LM. Improvements in quadriceps strength with regular seated exercise in the institutionalized elderly. *Archives of Physical Medicine and Rehabilitation* 1994;75:600–3.

114 Lichtenstein MJ, Shields SL, Shiavi RG, Burger MC. Exercise and balance in aged women: a pilot controlled clinical trial. *Archives of Physical Medicine and Rehabilitation* 1989;70:138–43.

115 Crilly RG, Willems DA, Trenholm KJ, Hayes KC, Delaquerriere-Richardson LF. Effect of exercise on postural sway in the elderly. *Gerontology* 1989;35:137–43.

116 Sherrington C, Lord SR. Home exercise to improve strength and walking velocity after hip fracture: a randomized controlled trial. *Archives of Physical Medicine and Rehabilitation* 1997;78:208–12.

117 Winter D. Overall principle of lower limb support during stance phase of gait. *Journal of Biomechanics* 1980;13:923–7.

118 Jette A, Lachman M, Giorgetti M, et al. Exercise – it's never too late: the strong-for-life programme. *American Journal of Public Health* 1999;89:66–72.

119 Jette AM, Harris BA, Sleeper L, et al. A home-based exercise programme for nondisabled older adults. *Journal of the American Geriatrics Society* 1996;44:644–9.

120 O'Reilly S, Muir K, Doherty M. Effectiveness of home exercise on pain and disability from osteoarthritis of the knee: a randomized controlled trial. *Annals of the Rheumatic Diseases* 1999;58:15–19.

121 Sashika H, Matsuba Y, Watanabe Y. Home programme of physical therapy: effect on disabilities of patients with total hip arthroplasty. *Archives of Physical Medicine and Rehabilitation* 1996;77:273–277.

122 Callaghan MJ, Oldham J, Hunt J. An evaluation of exercise regimes for patients with osteoarthritis of the knee: a single-blind randomized controlled trial. *Clinical Rehabilitation* 1995;9:213–18.

123 McMurdo ME, Johnstone R. A randomized controlled trial of a home exercise programme for elderly people with poor mobility. *Age and Ageing* 1995;24:425–18.

124 Buchner DM. Physical activity and quality of life in older adults (editorial). *Journal of the American Medical Association* 1997;277:64–6.

125 Hillsdon M, Thorogood M, Anstiss T, Morris J. Randomized controlled trials of physical activity promotion in free-living populations: a review. *Journal of Epidemiology and Community Health* 1995;49:448–53.

126 Kerschan K, Alacamlioglu Y, Kollmitzer J, et al. Functional impact of unvarying exercise programme in women after menopause. *American Journal of Physical Medicine and Rehabilitation* 1998;77:326–32.

9

Modifying the environment to prevent falls

This chapter outlines commonly suggested environmental modification strategies, and reviews the literature evaluating falls prevention programmes which have involved environmental modifications as individual interventions or as parts of multifaceted programmes. It discusses potential barriers to home modification, and issues related to hazard removal and design strategies for minimizing older people's risk of falling in public places. Approaches for addressing environmental risk factors within institutions are discussed in Chapter 12.

Environmental modification strategies

Table 6.1 presents the range of environmental falls risk factors that have been suggested in the literature. Table 9.1 lists these risk factors and outlines potential solutions.

Environmental modification as an individual intervention

Environmental modification is seen by many as an attractive falls prevention strategy. The homes of most older people have many environmental hazards [1, 2], and the majority of these are amenable to modification. Correction and/or removal of these hazards is a one-off intervention that can be carried out relatively cheaply. Indeed, cost-effectiveness modelling [3] has predicted that spending $244 per person on a programme involving home assessment by an occupational therapist and subsequent modifications, would save $92 per person and $916 per fall prevented, over a 10-year period. However, this study assumes that 25% of falls could be prevented by such a programme. Reductions of this magnitude have yet to be demonstrated in controlled studies.

There have now been two controlled clinical trials of home assessment and modification [4, 5] but only one of these [5] reported falls as an outcome measure. This study by Cumming et al. [5] was conducted among 530 community-dwellers, most of whom had been recently hospitalized. The intervention group received a home visit by an occupational therapist, who assessed the home for environmental

Table 9.1. Possible strategies to address environmental hazards

Risk factor	Solution
General	
Lighting (too low, excessive glare, uneven)	Ensure even, high, nonglare levels of illumination
	Use of night lights
Slippery floor surfaces	Nonslip floor surfaces
	Avoid excessive use of floor polish
Loose rugs	Removal or fixing down of loose rugs
Upended carpet edges	Repair of upended carpet edges and other uneven floor coverings
Raised door sills	Modification
Obstructed walkways	Clear walkways obstructed by furniture or other objects
Cord across walkways	Change cord path
Shelves or cupboards too high or too low	Avoid use of shelves or cupboards which are very high or low
Spilt liquids	Wipe up spilt liquids immediately
Pets	Take care with pets
	Training or restraint of dangerous pets
Furniture	
Low chairs	Chair raisers
Low or elevated bed height	Bed blocks or leg modification
Unstable furniture	Repair or removal of unstable furniture
Use of ladders and step ladders	Avoid use of ladders and stepladders
Bathroom/ toilet/ laundry	
Lack of grab rails: shower/bathtub/toilet	Installation of grab rails: shower/bathtub/toilet
Hob on shower recess	Removal of hob on shower recess
	Shower outside of shower recess area on a chair
Low toilet seat	Toilet seat raisers
Outdoor toilet	Use of commode instead of outdoor toilet
Slippery surfaces	Use of nonslip mats and strips
Use of bath oils	Avoid use of bath oils
Stairs	
No or inadequate handrails	Installation of appropriate handrails
Noncontrasting steps	Contrasting strips on step treads
Stairs too steep, tread too narrow	Modification of stairs

Table 9.1. (*cont.*)

Risk factor	Solution
Distracting surroundings	Modification of surrounding design
Unmodifiable stairs or individual unable to manage stairs	Installation of ramps
Outdoors	
Sloping, slippery, obstructed or uneven pathways, ramps and stairways	Redesign or modify pathways, ramps and stairways
Brief cycles in traffic lights	Longer cycles in traffic lights
Crowds	Care in crowds
	Use of walking aid to highlight frailty
Certain weather conditions (leaves, snow, ice, rain)	Removal of fallen leaves, water, snow, ice
	Care in dangerous weather conditions
Lack of places to rest	More places to rest provided
Unsafe garbage bin use	Redesign or provide assistance with garbage bins

hazards and facilitated any necessary home modifications. There was a significant reduction in the rate of falls among those who had fallen in the year prior to the study. In fact, the relative risk reduction was 35%. However, the effect on those who had not previously fallen was not significant. In addition, this study actually found a reduction in falls outside the home. As discussed by the authors, this suggests that the home modifications may not have been the major factor in the reduction in falls rates. Other aspects of the occupational therapy intervention, which included advice on footwear and behaviour, may have played an important role. This issue requires further investigation.

The second, smaller, study also involved an assessment by an occupational therapist, but did not report such encouraging findings. In this study of 167 older people, those found to require home modification and/or community services were randomized into either a group which had the occupational therapist's recommendations carried out, or a group which did not. At the 6-month follow-up, no differences were found on measures of health, mood, morale, life satisfaction or activities of daily living between the groups.

Three noncontrolled studies have shown positive effects of home assessment and modification programmes aimed at the general population of older people. One programme [6] involved assessment of the homes of older volunteers by 'home safety advisers', subsidized floor treatments (with nonslip material) and grab rail installation. Twelve months after the modifications, the 305 people who agreed to have modifications (90% of those visited) reported a 58% reduction in the number of falls experienced in the preceding 12 months. The results of this study should be viewed with some caution [7] due to the lack of a control group or investigator blinding and the use of volunteer subjects. Ytterstad [8] conducted a community-based programme in Norway which involved environmental assessment and modification, and promotion of safe footwear use in winter. They found decreased rates of fractures from falls in the intervention municipality and a rise in fracture rates in a reference city where the programme was not carried out. Plautz et al. [9] evaluated an intervention that involved home safety assessments and modifications such as removing clutter, installing hand rails, grab bars and nonskid strips and securing rugs and electrical cords. This involved an average of 10-person hours of unskilled labour and $93 worth of materials. Reported falls for the 6 months after the intervention were reduced by 60% compared with the 6 months prior to the intervention.

While there is some evidence supporting the role of home modification in falls prevention, much more investigation is required. It may also be that home assessment and modification have a greater role to play among more disabled individuals [10, 11]. Indeed an appropriate environment may make the difference between someone being able or not able to complete a functional task (such as taking a shower). If a person has only marginal ability to complete such a task, the appropriate modifications may also greatly enhance their safety. Indeed, the randomized controlled trial by Cumming et al. [5] showed that home visits were most effective in preventing falls among those who had previously fallen.

Environmental modification in multifactorial programmes

Although simple environmental modification interventions seem appealing as a falls prevention strategy, several authors have cautioned against the widespread implementation of this approach as a public health strategy [10, 12]. This strategy ignores the fact that falls result from an interaction between intrinsic (e.g. decreased balance control) and extrinsic (e.g. environmental hazard) factors. For example, a person who falls after tripping on an uneven piece of carpet is likely to do so because of decreased ability to recover from such an event, whereas a person with good recovery skills would be less likely to fall in this situation. While fixing the carpet may have prevented this particular fall, this 'faller' is likely to fall again when encountering another relatively trivial hazard. It is therefore likely that this person will gain greater overall benefits from interventions designed to address balance recovery skills as well.

A number of multifaceted falls prevention strategies including both intrinsic and extrinsic components have now been assessed with randomized controlled trials.

As is outlined in Chapter 15, several of these have been found to be effective [13–16] although others have not [17–19]. However, following pooling of data from some of these trials, the Cochrane review of falls prevention strategies concluded that 'an intervention in which older people are assessed by a health professional trained to identify intrinsic and environmental risk factors is likely to reduce the number of people sustaining falls (OR 0.79; 95% CI 0.65 to 0.96)' [20].

Unfortunately, the design of the multifaceted studies conducted to date does not allow assessment of the effects of individual strategies or their relative contributions to the success or otherwise of the various approaches. Further, these studies have involved a diverse array of interventions and differing degrees of emphasis on environmental aspects, which makes comparison between studies difficult. Nevertheless, multifaceted approaches to falls prevention appear to offer good scope for preventing falls in older people.

Barriers to environmental modification

Compliance with suggested modifications is a key issue for successful implementation of environmental falls prevention strategies. Studies have reported compliance rates for home and lifestyle safety modifications ranging from 22% [21] to 90% [6].

There are a number of potential barriers to a person adopting recommended environmental modifications. It has been reported that recommendations made by health professionals to reduce home hazards such as moving furniture, tacking down carpets or improving lighting are generally not welcomed by older people [22]. This may be because many older people are concerned about the possible stigmatizing effects of safety measures, and may feel that their own and others' views of their health and independence are being challenged [23]. Education programmes may assist in overcoming this barrier, as there is some evidence that compared with individual approaches, group education can increase the likelihood of compliance in adopting home modifications, especially with low-cost interventions [24].

Low financial status of older people is another limiting factor in implementing home modifications [23]. Community programmes which provide subsidized housing modifications to older people on low incomes offer a means of addressing this potential barrier. For example, the low intervention cost to participants is likely to have contributed to the high take-up rate of suggested modifications (90%) in the Thompson study [6].

Public places and design issues

The issue of how to design and build public environments and buildings in ways to accommodate the needs of older people is becoming more important as the world's population ages [25]. Environments should be designed to safely accommodate the needs of a range of users (i.e. with a range of physical abilities) in a range of different weather conditions.

Possible interventions in public places include: better design and maintenance of pavements and other surfaces, prevention of excessive accumulation of ice and snow, prompt cleaning up of spilt liquids, widespread implementation of contrasting edges on stairs, and increased provision of resting places and grab rails. The effects of such interventions are difficult to assess but implementation of ongoing falls surveillance by public authorities as suggested by Sattin [26] should assist in this process.

Garner [27] has outlined a range of strategies by which local governments can minimize the risk of falls in the community. She proposes two checklists for identifying hazards that warrant modification. The first is for assessing the adequacy of footpaths (including design, materials, construction, condition, obstructions and maintenance), steps and stairs, ramps and roadways. The second is for assessing safety in shopping centres, malls and arcades (including: assessments of entrances, steps, stairs and ramps, lighting, floor surfaces, furniture and fixtures, rest rooms, cleaning, lifts and escalators and policy and practice). The initiation and sustainability of this approach may require policy and design changes, and the establishment of access and safety committees to oversee this.

Changes to floor surfaces may have the potential to reduce falls injury rates. For example, there is some evidence that carpeted floors are associated with fewer falls injuries than vinyl floors [28]. More research is required to develop surfaces with optimal levels of friction for safety. These surfaces should have sufficient friction to minimize slips but not so much as to impede walking (i.e. to cause feet and shoes to drag on the surface). A number of countries are now developing building standards for slip resistance of surfaces to be used in different settings [29]. There are also calls for investigating better ways of dissipating the energy involved in a fall with energy-absorbing floors and surfaces [30]. These strategies mirror the approaches used successfully in automotive safety.

Conclusion

Environmental assessment and modification appears to contribute to the success of multifaceted falls prevention programmes. While this area remains underinvestigated as an individual falls prevention strategy, there is an indication of its potential effectiveness especially among high-risk populations. Solutions to potential barriers to an individual's adoption of proposed home modification such as education and financial assistance need to be considered and addressed. In addition, more attention should be paid to safety of public places and to ongoing falls data collection systems.

REFERENCES

1 Carter SE, Campbell EM, Sanson-Fisher RW, Redman S, Gillespie WJ. Environmental hazards in the homes of older people. *Age and Ageing* 1997;26:195–202.

2 Bray G. Falls risk factors for persons aged 65 years and over in New South Wales. Sydney: *Australian Bureau of Statistics*, 1995.

3 Smith RD, Widiatmoko D. The cost-effectiveness of home assessment and modification to reduce falls in the elderly. *Australian and New Zealand Journal of Public Health* 1998;22:436–40.

4 Liddle J, March L, Carfrae B, et al. Can occupational therapy intervention play a part in maintaining independence and quality of life in older people? A randomized controlled trial. *Australian and New Zealand Journal of Public Health* 1996;20:574–8.

5 Cumming R, Thomas M, Szonyi G, et al. Home visits by an occupational therapist for assessment and modification of environmental hazards: a randomized controlled trial of falls prevention. *Journal of the American Geriatrics Society* 1999;47:1397–1402.

6 Thompson PG: Preventing falls in the elderly at home: a community-based programme. *Medical Journal of Australia* 1996;164:530–2.

7 Cameron I, Kurrle S, Cumming R. Preventing falls in the elderly at home: a community-based programme (letter). *Medical Journal of Australia* 1996;165:459–60.

8 Ytterstad B. The Harstad injury prevention study: community based prevention of fall-fractures in the elderly evaluated by means of a hospital-based injury recording system in Norway. *Journal of Epidemiology and Community Health* 1996;50:551–8.

9 Plautz B, Beck DE, Selmar C, Radetsky M. Modifying the environment: a community-based injury-reduction programme for elderly residents. *American Journal of Preventive Medicine* 1996;12:33–8.

10 Campbell AJ, Borrie MJ, Spears GF, Jackson SL, Brown JS, Fitzgerald JL. Circumstances and consequences of falls experienced by a community population 70 years and over during a prospective study. *Age and Ageing* 1990;19:136–41.

11 Nevitt MC, Cummings SR, Kidd S, Black D. Risk factors for recurrent nonsyncopal falls. A prospective study. *Journal of the American Medical Association* 1989;261:2663–8.

12 Parker MJ, Twemlow TR, Pryor GA. Environmental hazards and hip fractures. *Age and Ageing* 1996;25:322–5.

13 Hornbrook MC, Stevens VJ, Wingfield DJ, Hollis JF, Greenlick MR, Ory MG. Preventing falls among community-dwelling older persons: results from a randomized trial. *Gerontologist* 1994;34:16–23.

14 Tinetti ME, Baker DI, McAvay G, et al. A multifactorial intervention to reduce the risk of falling among elderly people living in the community. *New England Journal of Medicine* 1994;331:821–7.

15 Wagner EH, LaCroix AZ, Grothaus L, et al. Preventing disability and falls in older adults: a population-based randomized trial. *American Journal of Public Health* 1994;84:1800–6.

16 Close J, Ellis M, Hooper R, Glucksman E, Jackson S, Swift C. Prevention of falls in the elderly trial (PROFET): a randomized controlled trial. *Lancet* 1999;353:93–97.

17 Fabacher D, Josephson K, Pietruszka F, Linderborn K, Morley J, Rubenstein L. An in-home preventive assessment programme for independent older adults. *Journal of the American Geriatrics Society* 1994;42:630–8.

18 Rubenstein LZ, Robbins AS, Josephson KR, Schulman BL, Osterweil D. The value of assessing falls in an elderly population. A randomized clinical trial. *Annals of Internal Medicine* 1990;113:308–16.

19 Vetter NJ, Lewis PA, Ford D. Can health visitors prevent fractures in elderly people? *British Medical Journal* 1992;304:888–90.

20 Gillespie LD, Gillespie WJ, Cumming R. Lamb SE, Rowe BH. Interventions for preventing falls in the elderly (Cochrane Review). The Cochrane Library, issue 3. Oxford: Update Software, 1999.

21 Ploeg J, Black ME, Hutchison BG, Walter SD, Scott EAF, Chambers LW. Personal, home and community safety promotion with community-dwelling elderly persons: response to a public health nurse intervention. *Canadian Journal of Public Health* 1994;85:188–91.

22 Isaacs B. Clinical and laboratory studies of falls in old people. Prospects for prevention. *Clinics in Geriatric Medicine* 1985;1:513–24.

23 Connell BR. Role of the environment in falls prevention. *Clinics in Geriatric Medicine* 1996;12:859–80.

24 Ryan JW, Spellbring AM. Implementing strategies to decrease risk of falls in older women. *Journal of Gerontological Nursing* 1996;22:25–31.

25 Gibson MJ, Andres RO, Isaacs B, Radebaugh T, Worm-Petersen J. The prevention of falls in later life. A report of the Kellogg International Work Group on the Prevention of Falls by the Elderly. *Danish Medical Bulletin* 1987;34:1–24.

26 Sattin RW. Falls among older persons: a public health perspective. *Annual Review of Public Health* 1992;13:489–508.

27 Garner E: *Preventing falls in public places: challenge and opportunity for local government.* Lismore, New South Wales: North Coast Public Health Unit, 1996.

28 Healey F. Does flooring type affect risk of injury in older in-patients? *Nursing Times* 1994;90:40–1.

29 Bowman R. What we must do to reduce pedestrian slips and falls. Third National Conference on Injury Prevention and Control, Brisbane, Australia, 1999.

30 Sattin RW, Rodriguez JG, DeVito CA, Wingo PA. Home environmental hazards and the risk of fall injury events among community-dwelling older persons. Study to Assess Falls Among the Elderly (SAFE) Group. *Journal of the American Geriatrics Society* 1998; 46: 669–76.

10

The role of footwear in falls prevention

Footwear has an important role in protecting the foot from extremes of tempera-ture, moisture and mechanical trauma. However, since the development and wide-spread popularity of 'fashion footwear' in the 1600s, the functional aspect of footwear has largely been supplanted by cosmetic requirements. In both men and women of all ages, shoe selection is primarily based on aesthetic considerations, many of which are incompatible with optimal function of the lower extremity [1]. This is of particular importance in older people, as certain types of footwear, by modifying the interface between the sole of the foot and the ground, may have a significant detrimental impact on postural stability.

Evidence to support the suggestion that shoes may influence postural stability can be derived from epidemiological investigations regarding falls in older people. Inappropriate styles of footwear, including shoes with high heels, narrow heels, slip-on shoes and worn slippers, have been implicated as a contributing factor in up to 50% of falls [2, 3]. Of particular interest, Finlay [4] reported that of 274 patients admitted to a geriatric unit and day hospital, just over half were wearing adequate footwear, and half of those who regularly wore slippers had a history of falling. One explanation for such a high prevalence of poor footwear habits may be that older people are generally unaware of the possible ramifications of inappropri-ate footwear, and base their footwear selection on comfort, rather than safety [4, 5].

Although there is some preliminary evidence to suggest an association between footwear and falls, the wearing of a particular style of shoe at the time of a fall does not necessarily confirm a direct causal relationship, as clearly there are a multitude of other factors involved. Nevertheless, it is probable that footwear may play a more significant role than the relatively small volume of literature would suggest, as foot-wear assessment is often overlooked in falls research. For example, a number of studies have attributed falls to environmental factors such as poorly maintained footpaths, walking up stairs or over uneven terrain, without considering the role of footwear in adapting to these environmental hazards [6–10]. Furthermore, the fact that a high proportion of falls occur when walking [9–11] suggests that footwear is

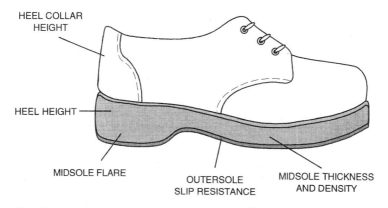

HEEL COLLAR
HEIGHT

HEEL HEIGHT

MIDSOLE FLARE

OUTERSOLE
SLIP RESISTANCE

MIDSOLE THICKNESS
AND DENSITY

Fig. 10.1.   Shoe features thought to influence postural stability in older people.

a 'hidden' variable which may contribute to a larger proportion of accidental falls than is widely recognized [4, 12].

A number of features of shoe design have been implicated as having an impact on postural stability (see Figure 10.1). The main features thought to play a role in affecting postural stability are heel height, the cushioning properties of the midsole, and the slip resistance of the outersole. Two additional features, the height of the heel collar and midsole geometry, have not been widely evaluated in the context of postural stability, but rather in relation to overuse injuries in sportspeople. However, given that a number of authors have recommended the wearing of 'high-top' boots or shoes with 'broad heels' as a means of improving stability in older people [4, 13–15], these features warrant further investigation. Each of these design components is discussed in more detail in the following sections.

Heel height

High heels first became widely used in the early 1600s, and despite minor fluctuations in their popularity, still remain a dominant feature in women's footwear [16, 17]. However, the use of heel elevation in footwear design is by no means restricted to women's shoes, as a number of boots worn by men also feature a raised heel (e.g. safety footwear, 'cowboy' boots). Research into the effects of heel elevation has tended to focus on postural and kinematic alterations, due to the proposed relationship between wearing high heels and the development of overuse symptoms in the foot, knee, hip and lower spine. These studies have revealed that heel elevation leads to a reduction in lumbar lordosis ('sway-back') [18–21], increased loading on the forefoot [22–26], alterations in the function of the big toe joint during the propulsive phase of gait [27, 28], decreased stride length [29], increased energy consumption [30], increased arch height [31] and altered motion of the ankle and knee joints [20, 25, 30, 32–37]. These alterations have generally been interpreted as detrimental to normal lower extremity function, however kinematic differences between inexperienced and experienced wearers of high heels suggests that some habituation occurs over time which may act to minimize these adverse effects [38–40].

A number of authors have suggested that the changes in function produced by high-heeled footwear may be responsible for instability and falling in older people [4, 12–14, 41, 42], and there is some epidemiological evidence to support this suggested relationship. In a prospective investigation of falls experienced by 100 older subjects, Gabell et al. [3] reported that the best predictor of multiple falling episodes was a history of wearing high-heeled footwear. However, all of the subjects with a history of high heel use were wearing a low-heeled shoe when they fell, suggesting that alterations in lower limb posture caused by years of high heel wearing may make the subject less stable when they change to wearing shoes with a lower heel profile.

High heels may contribute to instability and falling by affecting the position of the centre of mass and by altering the position of the foot when walking [25, 43]. Two recent reports have highlighted the detrimental impact of high heels on balance. Brecht et al. [44] reported that balance performance on a moving platform was significantly worse in a heeled cowboy boot compared with a tennis shoe, and suggested that heel elevation may make the wearer more susceptible to falling backwards. We have also found that balance ability in older women is detrimentally affected by high heels [45]. In our study, older women's balance was tested barefoot, in their own shoes and in high-heeled shoes. The worst balance performances occurred when women wore high-heeled shoes. These studies suggest that the wearing of high heels may be an unnecessary risk factor for falling in older people. However, further research needs to be undertaken to ascertain the optimum heel elevation for women's shoes, as many older women report that they feel safer in a 'slight' heel, and heel elevation may have some beneficial effects in older people with Parkinson's disease to facilitate forward propulsion [46].

Midsole cushioning

The use of expanded polymer foam materials in the construction of footwear midsoles is widely accepted as a means of enhancing the level of comfort the shoe can provide to the wearer, and as such is commonly recommended as a beneficial feature in footwear for older people [15, 47]. However, recent work by Robbins and colleagues suggests that the use of thick, soft materials in footwear midsoles leads to instability as the midsole material induces a state of 'sensory insulation', thereby reducing sensory input to the central nervous system regarding foot position [48].

To test this hypothesis, Robbins and colleagues have conducted a number of studies which have evaluated balance ability when older people wear footwear which varies according to the thickness and softness of the midsole material. These studies have found that shoes with thick, soft midsoles have a detrimental effect on the ability of older people to maintain balance when walking on a beam [48], to detect the position of their ankle joint when standing on different surface inclinations [49] and to detect the position of their foot when walking [50]. However, the beam walking method has been criticized as too dissimilar to normal overground walking [51], and the midsole materials used in these studies have been very soft. We recently found that midsole hardness was not associated with stability in older women; however, the materials used in the shoes in our study were not as soft as those used by Robbins et al. [52].

Nevertheless, the suggestion that soft shoes may have detrimental effects on balance has been supported by investigations by Finlay [4] who reported an association between wearing soft slippers and falls, and Frey and Kubasak [53], who found that a large number of older people who fell were wearing cushioned running shoes at the time. Furthermore, older subjects have been found to sway more on soft floors than hard floors [54], and we have shown that body sway when standing on foam is a good indicator of falls risk [55, 56]. It would therefore appear that the interaction between sensory feedback and stability proposed by Robbins and colleagues is plausible, and may contribute to falls among otherwise healthy older people. Large-scale prospective investigations are required to clarify whether a direct causal relationship exists between cushioning footwear and falls in older people, but it may be prudent to advise against the wearing of shoes with very soft soles unless there is a specific therapeutic need for extra cushioning.

Slip-resistance of footwear outersoles

Accidental falls caused by slipping are a common concern in older people, particularly in countries where snow- and ice-covered pavements cause a large number of injuries to older people during winter months [57, 58]. It has been estimated that over one million injuries caused by slipping are treated by hospitals in the UK every year [59], and the majority of these slipping incidents result in damage to the lumbar spine [60]. However, while a number of investigations have attributed falls in older people to slipping or tripping on unstable surfaces such as cracked paths, bathroom tiles or snow, few studies in the gerontology or rehabilitation literature have focused on the role of the outersole of the shoe in these accidents. Much of the work in this area has been performed in the context of occupational safety, due the high number of injuries in the workplace resulting from slipping on factory floors [59, 61].

In an attempt to decrease the high incidence of slipping accidents, considerable investigative effort has been directed towards the development of slip-resistant factory floors and footwear soles. However, progress towards a complete understanding of slip resistance is slow, due to the inability of testing apparatus to simulate accurately the wide variations in normal gait [60, 62] and the practical dilemma created by the fact that people walk over a wide range of surfaces during a normal day. Nevertheless, a number of authors have suggested that older people should be advised to avoid shoes with 'slippery' soles: the assumption being that a textured, slip-resistant sole may prevent slip-related accidents [4, 12–14, 41, 42]. Such a recommendation may not be appropriate in all situations, however, as a number of cases have been reported in which falls are attributed to 'excessive' slip-resistance of the shoe when walking on a pavement or performing a household task [3, 63]. However, it would appear that falls related to excessive slip-resistance are far less common than those resulting from inadequate slip-resistance.

Research reveals that slipping is most likely to occur when the heel first strikes the ground [57, 64, 65], and therefore, improving the grip of the sole at this point of the gait cycle may prevent slip-related falls. This may be achieved by constructing linear grooves in the outersole to disperse fluid from under the shoe [65], or by bevelling the rear part of the heel [66]. The effect of heel bevelling is shown in Figure 10.2. Although both these approaches have been found to be of benefit under experimental conditions, it remains to be seen whether such footwear modifications can help prevent slipping in older people. Thus, although some advances have been made in the understanding of slip-resistance in occupational safety research, difficulties arise in applying these findings to falls prevention in older people. Further research is therefore required to simulate the actual slipping event in an older person on a range of commonly encountered surfaces. Nevertheless, the widely reported recommendation of avoiding very slippery-soled shoes would appear to be appropriate in most cases.

Heel collar height

High heel collars are commonly found in safety footwear and in shoes designed for specific sporting activities such as football and basketball [67, 68]. Subsequently, much of the literature regarding the effects of heel collar height evaluates the ability of the shoe to prevent ankle sprains. Two main theories have been suggested to explain why high heel collars may be of benefit in ankle sprain prophylaxis. First, the mere presence of the material surrounding the ankle region is thought to provide mechanical stability to the ankle and subtalar joints in the frontal plane, such that rapid excursions of the foot into eversion or inversion are restricted by the shoe [69–71]. Second, the presence of the high heel collar may provide addi-

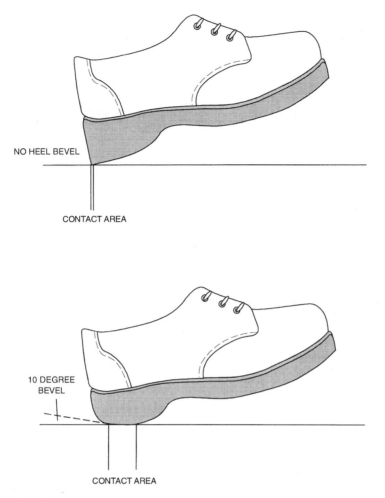

NO HEEL BEVEL

CONTACT AREA

10 DEGREE
BEVEL

CONTACT AREA

Fig. 10.2.   The effects of a heel bevel on slip-resistance. The greater contact area provided by the
bevel increases the coefficient of friction, thereby decreasing the likelihood of slipping
when the heel strikes the ground.

tional tactile stimulation, thereby improving proprioceptive feedback of ankle
position [67].

Stability around the heel is widely regarded as a desirable feature when recommending footwear for unstable older people, despite a lack of supporting evidence
[4, 13–15, 47]. We recently assessed the balance ability of older women when barefoot and in shoes with standard collar height (Oxford-style shoe) and a raised collar
height (eight-laced 'Doc Marten' boot). The results revealed that subjects performed better in the high collared shoe, presumably because the high heel-collar
provides greater ankle stability and increased proprioceptive feedback compared
with standard footwear [52].

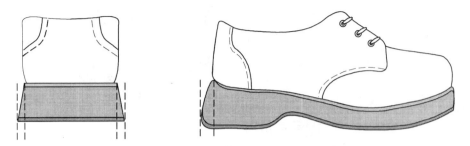

Fig. 10.3.   The midsole flare of a shoe.

The use of high heel collars as a means of improving stability in older people warrants further investigation, as both peripheral sensory loss [55] and ankle muscle weakness [72] have been found to contribute to falling. Given that ankle support has been found to improve mechanical stability and ankle position sense in younger people [70, 73], shoes with high collars may be able to compensate for age-associated declines in sensory and motor function of the foot and ankle. However, such shoes must not be too restrictive, as a certain amount of foot flexibility is required to adapt to uneven terrain when walking [74, 75].

Midsole flaring

The term 'midsole flare' refers to the difference between the width of the midsole at the level of the upper and its width at the level of the outersole (see Figure 10.3). A number of authors have suggested that a large midsole flare is of benefit to older people as it provides a broader base of support, thereby enhancing the stability of the shoe [4, 13–15, 41]. These recommendations appear to have been developed in response to the recognition of narrow heels (such as those found in most high-heeled footwear) provoking instability in older people. However, there are no studies in the literature which have directly evaluated the effect of midsole flaring on balance ability.

Theoretically, midsole flaring should improve mechanical stability by increasing the surface contact area of the shoe–ground interface [76, 77]. However, studies have also found that large midsole flares may make the foot pronate (roll inwards) more during gait [78, 79], and there is also the possibility that a large midsole flare may make the wearer susceptible to tripping by contacting the contralateral limb during the swing phase of gait. Whether these proposed detrimental effects of midsole flaring have significant ramifications for stability in older people is uncertain. Therefore, no absolute recommendations can yet be developed regarding the benefits or otherwise of midsole flaring in footwear for older people. However, our recent work suggests that impaired lateral stability is associated with falls [80], so

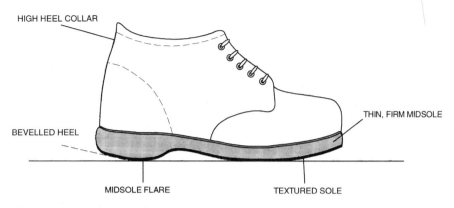

HIGH HEEL COLLAR

THIN, FIRM MIDSOLE

BEVELLED HEEL

MIDSOLE FLARE   TEXTURED SOLE

Fig. 10.4.   The theoretically optimal 'safe' shoe.

any attempt to improve the control of lateral movements of the centre of mass may be potentially beneficial.

Conclusion

Footwear may influence postural stability in either a beneficial or detrimental manner. Shoes alter the interface between the sole of the foot and the ground, both mechanically and neurophysiologically. Although many questions remain unanswered regarding the influence of specific design features on postural stability, it would seem reasonable to suggest that older people should be advised against the wearing of high-heeled shoes, shoes with very soft soles and shoes with slippery soles. Conversely, postural stability may be improved by the wearing of shoes with thin, flat, broad, bevelled heels constructed with a firm material, textured soles to improve traction, and possibly the addition of ankle support by the use of a high heel collar. The theoretically optimal 'safe' shoe for older people, is shown in Figure 10.4. Future research should address the effect of each of these variables on the stability of normal overground walking, and when navigating commonly encountered obstacles such as uneven ground, ramps and stairs.

REFERENCES

1 Coughlin MJ, Thompson FM. The high price of high-fashion footwear. *Instructional Course Lectures* 1995;44:371–7.

2 Barbieri E. Patient falls are not patient accidents. *Journal of Gerontological Nursing* 1983;9:165–73.

3 Gabell A, Simons MA, Nayak USL. Falls in the healthy elderly: predisposing causes. *Ergonomics* 1985;28:965–75.

4 Finlay OE. Footwear management in the elderly care programme. *Physiotherapy* 1986;72:172–8.

5 Dunne RG, Bergman AB, Rogers LW, Inglin B, Rivara FP. Elderly persons' attitudes towards footwear: a factor in preventing falls. *Public Health Reports* 1993;108(2):245–8.

6 Tinetti ME, Speechley M, Ginter SF. Risk factors for falls among elderly persons living in the community. *New England Journal of Medicine* 1988;319(26):1701–7.

7 Hindmarsh JJ, Estes EH. Falls in older persons: causes and interventions. *Archives of Internal Medicine* 1989;149:2217–22.

8 Campbell AJ, Borrie MJ, Spears GF, Jackson SL, Brown JS, Fitzgerald JL. Circumstances and consequences of falls experienced by a community population 70 years and over during a prospective study. *Age and Ageing* 1990;19:136–41.

9 Cali CM, Kiel DP. An epidemiologic study of fall-related fractures among institutionalized older people. *Journal of the American Geriatrics Society* 1995;43:1336–40.

10 Norton R, Campbell AJ, Lee-Joe T, Robinson E, Butler M. Circumstances of falls resulting in hip fractures among older people. *Journal of the American Geriatrics Society* 1997;45:1108–12.

11 Berg WP, Alessio HM, Mills EM, Tong C. Circumstances and consequences of falls in independent community-dwelling older adults. *Age and Ageing* 1997;26:261–8.

12 Rubenstein L, Robbins A, Schulman B, Rosada J, Osterweil D, Josephson K. Falls and instability in the elderly. *Journal of the American Geriatrics Society* 1988;36:266–78.

13 Edelstein JE. If the shoe fits: footwear considerations for the elderly. *Physical and Occupational Therapy in Geriatrics* 1987;5(4):1–16.

14 Edelstein JE. Foot care for the aging. *Physical Therapy* 1988;68:1882–6.

15 Sudarsky L. Geriatrics: gait disorders in the elderly. *New England Journal of Medicine* 1990;322:1441–6.

16 Frey CC, Thompson F, Smith J, Sanders M, Horstman H. American Orthopedic Foot and Ankle Society women's shoe survey. *Foot and Ankle* 1993;14:78–81.

17 Mitchell L. *Stepping out: three centuries of shoes*. Sydney: Powerhouse Publishing, 1997.

18 Bendix T, Sorenson SS, Klausen K. Lumbar curve, trunk muscles, and line of gravity with different heel heights. *Spine* 1984;9:223–7.

19 Opila KA, Wagner SS, Schiowitz S, Chen J. Postural alignment in barefoot and high-heeled stance. *Spine* 1988;13:542–7.

20 DeLateur BJ, Giaconi RM, Questad K, Ko M, Lehmann JF. Footwear and posture – compensatory strategies for heel height. *American Journal of Physical Medicine and Rehabilitation* 1991;70:246–54.

21 Franklin ME, Chenier TC, Brauninger L, Cook H, Harris S. Effect of positive heel inclination on posture. *Journal of Orthopedic and Sports Physical Therapy* 1995;21:94–9.

22 Gastwirth BW, O'Brien TD, Nelson RM, Manger DC, Kindig SA. An electrodynographic study of foot function in shoes of varing heel heights. *Journal of the American Podiatric Medical Association* 1991;81:463–72.

23 Snow RE, Williams KR, Holmes J. The effects of wearing high-heeled shoes on pedal pressures in women. *Foot and Ankle* 1992;13:85–92.

24 Corrigan JP, Moore DP, Stephens MM. Effect of heel height on forefoot loading. *Foot and Ankle* 1993;14:148–52.

25 Snow RE, Williams KR. High-heeled shoes: their effect on centre of mass position, posture, three dimensional kinematics, rearfoot motion and ground reaction forces. *Archives of Physical Medicine and Rehabilitation* 1994;75:568–76.

26 Nyska M, McCabe C, Linge K, Klenerman L. Plantar forefoot pressures during treadmill walking with high-heel and low-heel shoes. *Foot and Ankle International* 1996;17:662–6.

27 Sussman RE, D'Amico JC. The influence of the height of the heel on the first metatarsophalangeal joint. *Journal of the American Podiatric Medical Association* 1984;74:504–8.

28 McBride ID, Wyss UP, Cooke TD, Murphy L, Phillips J, Olney SJ. First metatarsophalangeal joint reaction forces during high-heel gait. *Foot and Ankle* 1991;11:282–8.

29 Merrifield HH. Female gait patterns in shoes with different heel heights. *Ergonomics* 1971;14:411–17.

30 Ebbeling CJ, Hamill J, Crussemeyer JA. Lower extremity mechanics and energy cost of walking in high-heeled shoes. *Journal of Orthopedic and Sports Physical Therapy* 1994;19:190–6.

31 Schwartz RP, Heath AL. Preliminary findings from a roentgenographic study of the influence of heel height and empirical shank curvature on osteo-articular relationships of the normal female foot. *Journal of Bone and Joint Surgery (Am)* 1959;46:324–34.

32 Gollnick PD, Tipton CM, Karpovich PV. Electromyographic study of walking on high heels. *Research Quarterly* 1964;35(Suppl):370–8.

33 Gehlsen G, Braatz SJ, Assmann N. Effects of heel height on knee rotation and gait. *Human Movement Science* 1986;5:149–55.

34 Soames RW, Evans AA. Female gait patterns: the influence of footwear. *Ergonomics* 1987;30:893–900.

35 Opila-Correia KA. Kinematics of high-heeled gait. *Archives of Physical Medicine and Rehabilitation* 1990;71:304–9.

36 Reinschmidt C, Nigg BM. Influence of heel height on ankle joint moments in running. *Medicine and Science in Sports and Exercise* 1995;27:410–6.

37 Kerrigan DC, Todd MK, Riley PO. Knee osteoarthritis and high-heeled shoes. *Lancet* 1998;351:1399–401.

38 Opila-Correia KA. Kinematics of high-heeled gait with consideration for age and experience of wearers. *Archives of Physical Medicine and Rehabilitation* 1990;71:905–9.

39 Lee KH, Matteliano A, Medige J, Smiehorowski T. Electromyographic changes of leg muscles with heel lift: therapeutic implications. *Archives of Physical Medicine and Rehabilitation* 1987;68:298–301.

40 Lee KH, Shieh JC, Matteliano A, Smiehorowski T. Electromyographic changes of leg muscles with heel lifts in women: therapeutic implications. *Archives of Physical Medicine and Rehabilitation* 1990;71:31–3.

41 Gibson MJ, Andres RO, Isaacs B, Radebaugh T, Worm-Petersen J. The prevention of falls in later life. *Danish Medical Bulletin* 1987;34 (Suppl 4):1–24.

42 Tinetti ME, Speechly M. Prevention of falls among the elderly. *New England Journal of Medicine* 1989;320:1055–9.

43 Adrian MJ, Karpovich PV. Foot instability during walking in shoes with high heels. *Research Quarterly* 1966;37:168–75.

44 Brecht JS, Chang MW, Price R, Lehmann J. Decreased balance performance in cowboy boots compared with tennis shoes. *Archives of Physical Medicine and Rehabilitation* 1995;76:940–6.

45 Lord SR, Bashford GM. Shoe characteristics and balance in older women. *Journal of the American Geriatrics Society* 1996;44:429–33.

46 Surdyk F, Kostyniuk P. Heel rise: an aid in ambulation for parkinsonian patients who lose their balance backward. *American Journal of Corrective Therapy* 1969;July:107.

47 Hogan-Budris J. Choosing foot materials for the elderly. *Topics in Geriatric Rehabilitation* 1992;7:49–61.

48 Robbins SE, Gouw GJ, McClaran J. Shoe sole thickness and hardness influence balance in older men. *Journal of the American Geriatrics Society* 1992;40:1089–94.

49 Robbins SE, Waked E, McClaran J. Proprioception and stability: foot position awareness as a function of age and footwear. *Age and Ageing* 1995;24:67–72.

50 Robbins SE, Waked E, Allard P, McClaran J, Krouglicof N. Foot position awareness in younger and older men: the influence of footwear sole properties. *Journal of the American Geriatrics Society* 1997;45:61–6.

51 Grabiner MD, Davis BL. Footwear and balance in older men (letter to the editor). *Journal of the American Geriatrics Society* 1993;41:1011–12.

52 Lord SR, Bashford GM, Howland A, Munro B. Effects of shoe collar height and sole density on balance in older women. *Journal of the American Geriatrics Society* 1999;47:681–4.

53 Frey CC, Kubasak M. Faulty footwear contributes to why seniors fall. *Biomechanics* 1998;5:45–7.

54 Redfern MS, Moore PL, Yarsky CM. The influence of flooring on standing balance among older persons. *Human Factors* 1997;39:445–55.

55 Lord SR, Clark RD, Webster IW. Physiological factors associated with falls in an elderly population. *Journal of the American Geriatrics Society* 1991;39:1194–200.

56 Lord SR, McLean D, Stathers G. Physiological factors associated with injurious falls in older people living in the community. *Gerontology* 1992;38:338–46.

57 Gronqvist R, Roine J, Jarvinen E, Korhonen E. An apparatus and a method for determining the slip resistance of shoes and floors by simulation of human foot motions. *Ergonomics* 1989;32:979–95.

58 Bjornstig U, Bjornstig J, Dahlgren A. Slipping on ice and snow: elderly women and young men are typical victims. *Accident Analysis and Prevention* 1997;29:211–5.

59 Manning DP, Ayers I, Jones C, Bruce M, Cohen K. The incidence of underfoot accidents during 1985 in a working population of 10 000 Merseyside people. *Journal of Occupational Accidents* 1988;10:121–30.

60 Manning DP. Slipping and the penalties inflicted generally by the law of gravitation. *Journal of Social and Occupational Medicine* 1988;38:123–7.

61 Bell J. Slip and fall accidents. *Occupational Health and Safety* 1995;December:40–1, 57.

62 Strandberg L. The effect of conditions underfoot on falling and over-exertion accidents. *Ergonomics* 1985;28:131–47.

63 Connell BR, Wolf SL. Environmental and behavioural circumstances associated with falls at home among healthy individuals. *Archives of Physical Medicine and Rehabilitation* 1997;78:179–86.

64 Perkins PJ, Wilson MP. Slip-resistance testing of shoes: new developments. *Ergonomics* 1983;26:73–82.

65 Tisserand M. Progress in the prevention of falls caused by slipping. *Ergonomics* 1985;28:1027–42.

66 Lloyd D, Stevenson MG. Measurement of slip resistance of shoes on floor surfaces, part 2. Effect of a bevelled heel. *Journal of Occupational Health and Safety* 1989;5:229–35.

67 Petrov O, Blocher K, Bradbury R. Footwear and ankle stability in the basketball player. *Clinics in Podiatric Medicine and Surgery* 1988;5:275–90.

68 Denton JA. Athletic shoes. In: Valmassy R, editor. *Clinical biomechanics of the lower extremities.* St Louis: Mosby, 1996:453–63.

69 Johnson G, Dowson D, Wrights V. A biomechanical approach to the design of football boots. *Journal of Biomechanics* 1976;9:581–5.

70 Ottaviani RA, Ashton-Miller JA, Kothari SU, Wojtys EM. Basketball shoe height and maximal muscular resistance to applied ankle inversion and eversion moments. *American Journal of Sports Medicine* 1995;23:418–23.

71 Stacoff A, Steger J, Stussi E, Reinschmidt C. Lateral stability in sideward cutting movements. *Medicine and Science in Sports and Exercise* 1996;28:350–8.

72 Whipple RH, Wolfson LI, Amerman PM. The relationship of knee and ankle weakness to falls in nursing home residents: an isokinetic study. *Journal of the American Geriatrics Society* 1987;35:13–20.

73 Robbins SE, Waked E, Rappel R. Ankle taping improves proprioception before and after exercise. *British Journal of Sports Medicine* 1995;29:242–7.

74 Matsusaka N. Control of the medial–lateral balance in walking. *Acta Orthopaedica Scandinavica* 1986;57:555–9.

75 Gauffin H, Tropp H. Postural control in single limb stance strategies for correction. *Journal of Human Movement Studies* 1994;26:267–78.

76 Hoogvliet P, Duyl WAV, Bakker JVD, Mulder PGH, Stam HJ. A model for the relation between the displacement of the ankle and the centre of pressure in the frontal plane, during one leg stance. *Gait and Posture* 1997;6:39–49.

77 Hoogvliet P, Duyl WAV, Bakker JVD, Mulder PGH, Stam HJ. Variations in foot breadth: effect on aspects of postural control during one-leg stance. *Archives of Physical Medicine and Rehabilitation* 1997;78:284–9.

78 Clarke TE, Frederick EC, Hamill CL. The effects of shoe design parameters on rearfoot control in running. *Medicine and Science in Sports and Exercise* 1983;15:376–81.

79 Nigg BM, Morlock M. The influence of lateral heel flare of running shoes on pronation and impact forces. *Medicine and Science in Sports and Exercise* 1987;19:294–302.

80 Lord SR, Rogers MW, Howland A, Fitzpatrick R. Lateral stability, sensorimotor function and falls in older people. *Journal of the American Geriatrics Society* 1999;47:1077–81.

Assistive devices

One quarter of older people use some sort of assistive device [1]. This chapter considers a range of devices which an older person may use to maximize physical ability and decrease risk of falling or of suffering an injury from a fall. Devices to be addressed include walking aids, other physical assistive devices, spectacles, hip protectors, aids to prevent 'long lies' and restraints. The potential impact of each of these devices on falls and/or falls injury is discussed.

Walking aids

Walking aids are commonly recommended to older people as a means of increasing their walking ability and decreasing their risk of falling. The prescription of a walking aid, however, is not a straightforward procedure. While appropriate for many older people, walking aids should ideally be prescribed by a health professional, after an assessment of the person's gait. Commonly used walking aids are outlined in Table 11.1.

Indications

The main indications for a walking aid are excessive pain on weight bearing, decreased leg muscle strength and control, instability, shortness of breath, poor vision and poor distal lower limb proprioception. These deficits may either be associated with acute events such as surgery or major illness, or with chronic conditions leading to a more gradual decline in physical abilities. Walking aids may have the additional benefit of marking frailty so that others take care when walking near the person using the aid in public. Some older people also report that an aid may be useful in self-defence [2].

A walking aid can reduce pain experienced in weight bearing by decreasing the load on the joints of the lower limbs as up to half the body weight can be taken through a walking aid [3]. This may be of great benefit to people suffering from arthritis, and following lower limb fractures or joint replacements.

A walking aid may assist in maximizing the safety and independence of gait for

Table 11.1. Types of walking aids

Sticks
Single (wooden or metal)
Quad (four-pronged)

Crutches
Axillary (fit under axilla, weight taken on hands)
Canadian (weight taken through hands and forearms)
Forearm support

Frames
Forearm support (large wheeled frames on which the forearms are placed)
Rollator (smaller wheeled frames which are pushed using hands)
Pick-up (without wheels, the person picks up the frame and places it in front of them and then steps up to it)

---

a person who has difficulty generating and/or coordinating appropriate force in the lower limb musculature. Substantial extensor torque is required to support the body weight against gravity. This extension of the hip, knee and ankle during stance phase is central to independent gait [4] and has been described as an essential component of walking [5]. Use of a walking aid can compensate for an inability to keep the leg extended against gravity. The hip abductors also play a crucial role in walking; large amounts of hip abductor muscle contraction are required during stance phase to keep the pelvis horizontal. The use of a walking aid decreases the hip abductor muscle force requirements [3], especially if held in the contralateral hand [6]. The ankle plantarflexors are also very important in normal walking, primarily in generating eccentric force to restrain forward motion of the lower limb [7]. A contralateral walking stick can compensate for poor plantarflexor muscle strength or control [3, 8]. In these instances the aid will enable the person to compensate for this lack of lower limb strength and/or control by using the upper limb musculature.

If a person is unsteady while standing and walking they may also benefit from a walking aid. A walking stick can effectively increase their base of support [3], which may increase stability, and may also assist the person to feel more confident. Walking with a frame allows the person to use their upper limbs to assist the lower limbs in maintaining an upright posture, thereby compensating for poor postural control.

People with chronic airflow limitation and other respiratory or cardiac conditions leading to a shortness of breath may find a wheeled walking aid useful. Studies have shown that such a walking aid increases the distance that people with chronic airflow limitation can walk [9, 10].

A walking aid may also be of assistance when sensory information is impaired, such as following amputation or peripheral nerve damage [3], or in individuals with poor vision. Jeka and Lackner [11] have shown that light finger touch of a firm support can dramatically increase standing stability in young people, and in a recent study we have found that such tactile information is also beneficial for balance in older people who fall and people with diabetic neuropathy [12]. This indicates that in addition to providing a mechanical support, a walking aid can provide the person with information about their position in and movement through the environment.

Prescription principles

A walking aid is best prescribed by a health professional after assessment of gait, muscle strength, balance and pain. Older people should be discouraged from purchasing or borrowing walking aids without such an assessment [13]. Several authors have suggested methods for prescribing walking aids [14–17]. As different walking aids have different characteristics, the person's abilities and environment need to be taken into account when prescribing an aid. For example, a rollator frame may be difficult to manoeuvre in a small bathroom, a pick-up frame may be unsafe for someone who is unable to stand unsupported while moving it forwards and the stability of a quad stick may encourage a person to bear excessive weight through their upper limb. A person may also need to use different aids when walking outdoors than when indoors [18].

An individual's use of a walking aid should be reviewed at regular intervals as their needs are likely to change over time. A further assessment may reveal that the person no longer needs the aid or requires a different aid. The user must also be taught how to maintain the aid. For example, worn ferrules are commonly found on walking aids used in the community [13]. These pose an easily avoidable risk to the user.

A large number of walking aids are commercially available. These vary considerably on a number of aspects of their design, which enables further tailoring of the aid to an individual's needs. For example, when choosing a walking frame, aspects to consider include: weight, base area, manoeuvrability, handle design, foldability, brake design and attachments such as seats and baskets [15]. A tray may also be a useful addition to a frame, enabling the individual to carry items independently [19]. The skill required to use a particular aid also should be considered. For example, attentional demands have been found to be greater with a pick-up frame than with a rollator frame [20]. This indicates the more complex nature of the task of walking with a pick-up frame and probably reflects its greater apparent variation from the biomechanical requirements of normal walking.

The height of a walking aid may also affect its usefulness. If a walking aid is too low it may cause excessive lateral flexion of the spine which may decrease gait efficiency and cause pain. If it is too high, the person may be required to elevate their shoulder to hold the aid which may also lead to pain. The usual height of an aid allows the elbow to be in 15–30 degrees of flexion. If the elbow is flexed more than 30 degrees (i.e. the aid is higher) the person is likely to put less weight on the aid. If the aid is lower the person will tend to put more weight on it [21, 22].

A walking aid should be prescribed after an assessment of the person's physical problems and analysis of the causes of these and the interaction of physical, environmental and psychosocial factors, rather than on a preconceived idea of what is appropriate for a certain condition [15, 23]. Creative thinking by the healthcare professional may also be required in walking aid prescription. For example, a person with Parkinson's disease who suffers from 'freezing' while walking, may benefit from a stick with a horizontal bar close to its distal end to either step over [24] or touch [25], or a frame with a piece of horizontal string which the person aims to kick.

Limitations

There are several limitations of and disadvantages to the use of walking aids. These can be summarized as: adverse effects on upper limbs, deterioration of motor function, energy consumption, social stigma and possible increased risk of falling.

Walking with an aid has the potential to cause pain in the joints of the arm, particularly the shoulder. The upper limb joints are subject to unaccustomed compressive forces as a result of bearing weight on the arms. In addition, Crosbie and Nicol have found that the upper limb musculature is required to generate large amounts of force [26, 27], which also leads to compressive forces over joints. However, they also found that the loads imposed on the upper limbs can be reduced by modifications to the gait pattern used when walking with crutches ('alternate step' rather than 'step to') [26] and by a modification to crutch design (by angling and retracting the crutch shaft to bring the arm closer to the trunk) [27].

As with any motor skill, walking involves the coordination of different muscle actions. It can be argued that walking with a walking aid is a fundamentally different skill from walking unaided. During aided gait, as the arms are assisting the legs in maintaining an upright position against gravity, the nature of the task is changed. The differing demands of the two tasks are reflected in the different ways the tasks are performed. For example, when walking with a frame the hip remains in a flexed position throughout the gait cycle [27], unlike unaided gait [28]. It is therefore possible that once an older person has learnt to walk with a walking aid, it may be difficult for them to walk unaided. They may need training and practice to relearn the skill of walking unaided [29]. In addition, if a person then becomes reliant on the use of a walking aid, they may actually be more unsafe when they attempt to stand, walk or reach outside of their base of support without hand support. This will interfere with their ability to carry out activities of daily living independently and is likely to increase their risk of falling.

Some people may be required by medical practitioners to fully unload a lower limb due to a complicated fracture or surgery. If the person is able, they may hop with crutches or a frame. When compared with unaided gait, this procedure has been associated with increased energy consumption, an increased heart rate [30, 31], and an increased oxygen cost [31, 32]. This increase appears to be greater for walking with a 'pick-up' frame than for walking with crutches [32]. This may put undue stress on the already compromised cardiovascular systems of some older people.

Some older people may also be reluctant to use a walking aid due to negative social stigma associated with the use of assistive devices [2, 33]. The health professional needs to be conscious of these issues when suggesting that an older person requires an aid.

While it seems likely that the appropriate use of a walking aid could contribute to falls prevention, no study has yet demonstrated that this is the case. In fact, the use of walking aids has been associated with an increased risk of falling [34–36]. As some people may fall as a direct consequence of the use of an aid (e.g. by tripping over the aid, catching the aid on furniture, or as a result of a poorly maintained aid) care needs to be taken to minimize this. However, it seems likely that most of these people are actually falling because of impaired gait and the use of a walking aid is merely an indicator of this impairment.

Alternatives

Use of a walking aid basically enables the individual to continue to walk despite problems such as excessive pain, decreased muscle strength and poor balance. The walking aid serves to compensate for these problems. Other strategies (such as exercise programmes, motor training, pain relief) to address these problems should be considered instead of, or in addition to, the prescription of the aid. As was outlined in Chapter 8, older people generally have much potential to improve their strength, balance and gait.

Other physical assistive devices

A number of other devices have been designed to assist the older person to interact with their environment more safely and easily, and thus maintain independence. Assistive devices can be classified as those designed to assist with: physical disabilities, hearing impairments, visual impairments, tactile impairments, and cognitive impairments [37]. Physical devices include: bath seats and benches, handheld showers, toilet surrounds, modified cutlery [38], modified cooking equipment [39], shower chairs, bath mats [40], orthoses [41–43], bath treads and lifts [44], long-handled shoehorns, reachers, sponges, sock-aids [45], remote control for televisions, cordless phones [46], lift chairs [46, 47], adaptive shoelaces [48], wheelchairs and motorized scooters [18].

Several authors have outlined prescription principles for physical assistive devices [16, 44, 48, 49]. Many assistive devices are best prescribed by an occupational therapist following a visit to the person's home to assess their needs in their own environment [45, 50]. Indeed, even people with cognitive impairments have the potential to increase their use of assistive devices after intervention from an occupational therapist [38].

Several clinical trials have now found value in the prescription and use of assistive devices. Hart et al. [39] conducted a randomized controlled trial of 79 community-dwellers aged 85 and over with some disability but not using any assistive devices prior to the study intervention. Following assessment by an occupational therapist, subjects in the intervention group were issued with a raised toilet seat, a teapot tipper, a tap turner, a shoehorn and elastic laces and a double-handled saucepan. Observed degree of difficulty in completing relevant tasks was subsequently reduced. In a randomized controlled trial of a home visit from an occupational therapist after discharge from hospital among people who had suffered a stroke, Corr and Bayer [51] found that the intervention group who used more aids were less likely to be readmitted to hospital.

Further investigation is required to assess the effects of these improvements on falls. Promisingly, occupational therapy assessment and provision of appropriate aids was a key component of one recent randomized controlled trial which showed a significant decrease in falls among people who had previously presented to the Emergency Department following a fall [52].

Spectacles

As indicated in Chapter 3, poor vision is prevalent in older people and constitutes a significant independent risk factor for falling. Spectacles are therefore essential for most older people, and it is important that they provide the optimal visual correction for each individual. To ensure that vision is maximized, it is important for older people to have regular eye examinations (at least every 2 years) so that correct prescription spectacles can be provided. It is also important to advise older people to actually wear their glasses and to keep them clean. For those with cataracts and others susceptible to glare, wearing prescription sunglasses and/or a hat with a brim when outside can dramatically enhance vision.

Another unnecessary visual hazard for older people is bi- or multifocal spectacles. These are prescribed for presbyopia – the most common visual condition associated with ageing. Presbyopia is a refractive condition that occurs when the crystalline lens–ciliary body complex loses the flexibility it requires to focus on distant as well as near objects [53]. In essence they are designed so that the lower sections can be used for viewing close objects and the top section for viewing more distant objects. Tri- and multifocal glasses have intermediate steps for mid-working distances. Multiple focal spectacles have definite benefits as they are convenient and are advantageous for tasks that require frequent changes to visual working distances such as cooking and driving. However, bifocal and multifocal glasses also have disadvantages. One limitation of bifocals is optical defects such as prismatic jump at the top of the reading segment [54].

The lower lenses of bifocal glasses also blur middle distance objects in the lower visual field, and this could represent a significant problem for older people. In a recently completed study involving 156 community-dwelling older people, we found that those who wore bi- and multifocals performed significantly worse on tests of depth perception and the edge contrast sensitivity which involved viewing middle distance objects through the bottom section of their spectacles [55]. This has practical implications, in that as we walk we detect obstacles (footpath cracks and misalignments, gutters and steps) at about two steps ahead. Clearly, if such objects can only be viewed through the lower spectacle section designed for near vision, they will not be in sharp focus. Whereas persons in middle age may be able to compensate for the elective disability that bifocals provide, older persons – particularly those who also have impairments of lower limb sensation, strength, coordination and balance – may not be able to recover from a trip or stumble over an unseen object. There is an easy alternative to multiple focal spectacles, two pairs of spectacles – one for reading and one for walking.

Hip protectors

It may be possible to decrease the likelihood that a fall will result in a fracture by changing the interaction between the faller and the surface on which they fall. This can be undertaken by modifying the surface onto which the person falls (as discussed previously) or by placing a barrier between the person and the hard surface onto which they fall. Hip protectors are designed to fulfil this latter role.

Hip protectors are worn by the individual and are designed both to absorb energy and to transfer load from the bone to the surrounding soft tissues [56]. The original hip protectors designed in Denmark [57] have a firm outer shell and an inner foam section. Another version is made of dense plastic without an outer shell [58]. The protector is either removable and fits into pockets in special underwear or nonremovable and built into underwear. The Danish model was tested in a randomized controlled study among 701 residents of a nursing home [57]. The risk of fracture was significantly decreased in the intervention group (relative risk 0.44). Interestingly, although eight members of the intervention group suffered hip fractures, none were wearing the hip protectors at the time of fracture. A further study in Sweden [59] tested a different model of hip protector and also found a decreased fracture rate among residents of a randomly selected nursing home who were offered hip protectors compared with a control nursing home (relative risk 0.33).

A hip protector will obviously not be effective in preventing a fracture if is not worn at the time of a fall. Studies based in nursing homes reported that 24–63% [57, 59–61] of people in the treatment group wore their hip protectors regularly. Such a study has yet to be completed among community-dwellers. Comfort is a key factor in compliance [62, 63]. The hip protector must also be correctly positioned to be effective. To maximize the chance of this, a person requires several pairs of underwear suitable to accommodate the device. This may involve additional expense and/or frequent washing. Incontinence makes the wearing of hip protectors more difficult [63], and may mean that frequent changes of underwear are required. Upper limb weakness may also mean that hip protectors are harder to apply [63].

No study investigating the effect of hip protectors among community-dwellers has yet been published. Several studies are currently investigating the feasibility of the use of hip protectors in this population [58]. It should also be noted that hip protectors may not necessarily decrease the risk of other fractures; there is a recent report of a person suffering a pelvic fracture from a fall while wearing a hip protector [64].

The design of hip protectors represents a balance between efficacy and comfort. After testing the Danish hip protectors in a laboratory setting, Mills [56] concludes that they would be more effective with a thicker foam inner section and a stiffer outer shell. Hip protectors appear to be a useful fracture prevention strategy. However, further investigation of their efficacy, optimal design, compliance issues and their use among community-dwellers is required.

Aids to prevent 'long lies'

Up to half of all older people who fall without suffering injuries are unable to get up from the floor unaided [65]. As well as additional emotional distress, this can result in a number of serious medical problems, as outlined in Chapter 1. If possible, older people should be taught how to get up off the floor [66].

For persons unable to get up from the floor independently, one way of preventing long lies is the use of personal alarm systems. These involve the older person having an alert button within reach at all times, i.e. worn on a cord around the neck or kept in a pocket. If the person falls and requires assistance, the alarm allows them to notify those nearby and/or an operator who can arrange for appropriate assistance to be provided. Although not evaluated in research trials, many older people and their families report feeling reassured once such a system is installed. Unfortunately, the cost of these systems may be prohibitive to some older people. Less costly alternatives are mobile or cordless phones carried by the older person at all times.

If an older person is at risk of not being able to get off the floor following a fall, steps should also be taken to minimize the consequences of the time spent on the floor [67]. For example, a blanket can be kept on or near the floor in commonly used rooms of the house to prevent hypothermia while waiting for help to arrive [66].

Restraints

Physical restraints can be used to prevent a person falling. They are commonly used in institutional settings, primarily to limit harm from unsteadiness while walking, disruptive behaviour or wandering [68]. Many items and actions constitute restraint including: cuffs to stop the person moving one or more limbs by fixing them to an object, jackets to stop a person sitting up in bed or getting out of a chair, tables to stop the person getting out of a chair, bed rails, use of low chairs or beds to prevent the person standing up, as well as certain medications (chemical restraints).

The use of restraints is highly controversial. It is clear that the widespread use of restraints impinges on the person's autonomy and personal freedom with associated philosophical and legal ramifications. Inappropriate restraint use could also lead to a deterioration in motor functioning if physical activity levels are insufficient to maintain muscle strength. Some restraints may also increase the risk of injury (e.g. skin damage from cuff, fall while attempting to climb over bedrail). Several authors have found that the use of restraints does not even decrease the risk of falls injury [69–72].

In recent years programmes have been introduced and legislation has been enacted in many countries to minimize the use of restraints. Werner et al. [73] reported the successful removal of restraints in 92% of previously restrained residents in a long-term care setting. Similarly, Levine et al. [74] reported being able to reduce the prevalence of physical restraint use in a large nursing facility from 39% to 4% over a 3-year period without a change in the rate of falls or accident-related injuries. Restraint use can be reduced more easily in purpose-built facilities where the person is safe to walk around freely. In poorly designed facilities people may be restrained to prevent them becoming lost, or injuring themselves on unsafe equipment or other environmental factors.

However, there is also evidence that in certain circumstances, restraints may play a role in falls injury prevention [75]. For example, a restraint may be required to prevent an older person with acute confusion who has already suffered several falls and is unaware that he or she is at a high risk of falling from walking unsupervised. If restraints are necessary in a particular setting they should be used with great caution. There should be strict protocols for when restraints may be used and who is able to authorize such use. Restraints should not be used routinely but rather prescribed for particular individuals for short time periods with regular review. A range of restraining devices should be available, optimally designed to minimize the risk to the patient. All alternatives should be fully investigated prior to the prescription of a restraint.

Conclusion

A large range of assistive devices have been discussed in this chapter. These impact either positively or negatively on the physical abilities or safety of older people. However, for each type of assistive device discussed above, more research is required to clarify its potential contribution to falls and fracture prevention. Each of these assistive devices should be carefully prescribed following assessment of the person's abilities and needs.

REFERENCES

1 Watts J, Erickson A, Houde L, Wilson E, Maynard M. Assistive device use among the elderly: a national data-based survey. *Physical and Occupational Therapy in Geriatics* 1996; 14:1–18.

2 Aminzadeh F, Edwards N. Exploring seniors' views on the use of assistive devices in fall prevention. *Public Health Nursing* 1998;15:297–304.

3 Deathe A, Hayes K, Winter D. The biomechanics of canes, crutches and walkers. *Critical Reviews in Physical and Rehabilitation Medicine* 1993;5:15–29.

4 Winter D. Overall principle of lower limb support during stance phase of gait. *Journal of Biomechanics* 1980;13:923–7.

5 Carr J, Shepherd R. *A motor relearning programme for stroke*, 2nd ed. London: Heinemann, 1987.

6 Neumann D. Hip abductor muscle activity as subjects with hip prostheses walk with different methods of using a cane. *Physical Therapy* 1998;78:490–501.

7 Sutherland D, Cooper C, Daniel D. The role of the ankle plantar flexors in normal walking. *Journal of Bone and Joint Surgery (Am)* 1980;62:354–63.

8 Moseley A, Wales A, Herbert R, Schurr K, Moore S. Observation and analysis of hemiplegic gait: stance phase. *Australian Journal of Physiotherapy* 1993;39:259–67.

9 Wesmiller S, Hoffman L. Assistive device for ambulation in oxygen-dependent patients with COPD. *Journal of Cardiopulmonary Rehabilitation* 1994;14:122–6.

10 Honeyman P, Barr P, Stubbing D. Effect of a walking aid on disability, oxygenation, and breathlessness in patients with chronic airflow limitation. *Journal of Cardiopulmonary Rehabilitation* 1996;16:63–7.

11 Jeka JJ, Lackner JR. Fingertip contact influences human postural control. *Experimental Brain Research* 1994;100:495–502.

12 Rogers M, Wardman D, Lord S, Fitzpatrick R. Tactile sensory input improves stability during standing in normal subjects and those with lower-limb sensory loss. (Paper in preparation.)

13 Simpson C, Pirrie L. Walking aids: a survey of suitability and supply. *Physiotherapy* 1991;77:231–4.

14 Breuer J. Assistive devices and adapted equipment for ambulation programmes for geriatric patients. *Physical & Occupational Therapy in Geriatrics* 1981;1:51–77.

15 Hall J, Clarke A, Harrison R. Guidelines for prescription of walking frames. *Physiotherapy* 1990;76:118–20.

16 Holliday P, Fernie G. Assistive devices: aids to independence. In: Pickles B, Compton A, Cott C, et al., editors. *Physiotherapy with older people.* London: Saunders, 1995:360–81.

17 Prajapati C, Watkins C, Cullen H, Orugun O, King D, Rowe J. The 'S' test: a preliminary study of an instrument for selecting the most appropriate mobility aid. *Clinical Rehabilitation* 1996;10:314–18.

18 York J. Mobility methods selected for use in home and community environments. *Physical Therapy* 1989;69:736–47.

19 Farley R, Roy J. Equipment review: the Edinburgh Homewalker. Design and field trial. *British Journal of Occupational Therapy* 1996;59:22.

20 Wright D, Kemp T. The dual-task methodology and assessing the attentional demands of ambulation with walking devices. *Physical Therapy* 1992;72:306–15.

21 Deathe AB, Pardo RD, Winter DA, Hayes KC, Russell-Smyth J. Stability of walking frames. *Journal of Rehabilitation Research and Development* 1996;33:30–5.

22 Lu CL, Yu B, Basford JR, Johnson ME, An KN. Influences of cane length on the stability of stroke patients. *Journal of Rehabilitation Research and Development* 1997;34:91–100.

23 Wilkin C. Pragmatics in the issuing of sticks and frames. *Physiotherapy* 1996;82:331–5.

24 Pearce J. A walking aid for parkinsonian patients (letter). *Lancet* 1993;342:62.

25 Blau J. Seymour stick (letter). *Lancet* 1993;342:250.

26 Crosbie W, Nicol A. Aided gait in rheumatoid arthritis following knee arthroplasty. *Archives of Physical Medicine and Rehabilitation* 1990;71:299–303.

27 Crosbie J. Kinematics of walking frame ambulation. *Clinical Biomechanics* 1993;8:31–6.

28 Winter DA, Patla AE, Frank JS, Walt SE. Biomechanical walking pattern changes in the fit and healthy elderly. *Physical Therapy* 1990;70:340–7.

29 Carr J, Shepherd R. *Neurological rehabilitation: optimizing motor performance.* Oxford: Butterworth-Heinemann, 1998.

30 Baruch I, Mossberg K. Heart-rate response of elderly women to nonweight-bearing ambulation with a walker. *Physical Therapy* 1983;63:1782–7.

31 Annesley A, Almada-Norfleet M, Arnall D, Cornwall M. Energy expenditure of ambulation using the Sure-Gait crutch and the standard axillary crutch. *Physical Therapy* 1990;70:18–23.

32 Holder C, Haskvitz E, Weltman A. The effects of assistive devices on the oxygen cost, cardiovascular stress, and perception of nonweight-bearing ambulation. *Journal of Orthopaedic and Sports Physical Therapy* 1993;18:537–42.

33 Rush KL, Ouellet LL. Mobility aids and the elderly client. *Journal of Gerontological Nursing* 1997;23:7–15.

34 Tinetti ME, Speechley M, Ginter SF. Risk factors for falls among elderly persons living in the community. *New England Journal of Medicine* 1988;319:1701–7.

35 Campbell AJ, Borrie MJ, Spears GF. Risk factors for falls in a community-based prospective study of people 70 years and older. *Journal of Gerontology* 1989;44:M112–17.

36 Kiely DK, Kiel DP, Burrows AB, Lipsitz LA. Identifying nursing home residents at risk for falling. *Journal of the American Geriatrics Society* 1998;46:551–5.

37 Mann W, Hurren D, Tomita M. Comparison of assistive device use and needs of home-based older persons with different impairments. *American Journal of Occupational Therapy* 1993;47:980–7.

38 Nochajski S, Tomita M, Mann W. The use and satisfaction with assistive devices by older persons with cognitive impairments: a pilot intervention study. *Topics in Geriatric Rehabilitation* 1996;12:38–53.

39 Hart D, Bowling A, Ellis M, Silman A. Locomotor disability in very elderly people: value of a programme for screening and provision of aids for daily living. *British Medical Journal* 1990;301:216–20.

40 Clemson L, Martin R. Usage and effectiveness of rails, bathing and toileting aids. *Occupational Therapy in Health Care* 1996;10:41–59.

41 Isakov E, Mizrahi J, Onna I, Susak Z. The control of genu recurvatum by combining the Swedish knee-cage and an ankle–foot brace. *Disability & Rehabilitation* 1992;14:187–91.

42 Berenter R, Kosai D. Various types of orthoses used in podiatry. *Clinics in Podiatric Medicine and Surgery* 1994;11:219–29.

43 Hesse S, Gahein-Sama A, Mauritz K-H. Technical aids in hemiparetic patients: prescription, costs and usage. *Clinical Rehabilitation* 1996;10:328–333.

44 Mann W, Hurren D, Tomita M, Charvat B. Use of assistive devices for bathing by elderly who are not institutionalised. *Occupational Therapy Journal of Research* 1996;16:261–86.

45 Finlayson M, Havixbeck K. A post-discharge study on the use of assistive devices. *Canadian Journal of Occupational Therapy* 1992;59:201–7.

46 Mann W, Hurren D, Tomita M. Assistive devices used by home-based elderly persons with arthritis. *American Journal of Occupational Therapy* 1995;49:810–20.

47 Munro B, Steele J, Bashford G, Ryan M, Britten N. A kinematic and kinetic analysis of the sit-to-stand transfer using an ejector chair: implications for elderly rheumatoid arthritic patients. *Journal of Biomechanics* 1998;31:263–71.

48 Schemm R, Gitlin L. How occupational therapists teach older patients to use bathing and dressing devices in rehabilitation. *American Journal of Occupational Therapy* 1998;52:276–82.

49 Gitlin L, Burgh D. Issuing assistive devices to older patients in rehabilitation: an exploratory study. *American Journal of Occupational Therapy* 1995;49:994–1000.

50 Clarke P, Gladman J. A survey of predischarge occupational therapy home assessment visits for stroke patients. *Clinical Rehabilitation* 1995;9:339–42.

51 Corr S, Bayer A. Occupational therapy for stroke patients after hospital discharge: a randomized controlled trial. *Clinical Rehabilitation* 1995;9:291–6.

52 Close J, Ellis M, Hooper R, Glucksman E, Jackson S, Swift C. Prevention of falls in the elderly trial (PROFET): a randomized controlled trial. *Lancet* 1999;353:93–7.

53 Patorgis C. Presbyopia. In: Amos J, editor. *Diagnosis and management in vision care.* Stoneham, UK: Butterworth, 1987.

54 El-Arabi M, Rashed O. Bifocal glasses. Optical principles and defects. *Bulletin of the Ophthalmological Society of Egypt* 1971;64:237–48.

55 Lord S, Matters B, Howland A. Visual risk factors for falls in older people. In: Proceedings of Aged Care Australia and Australian Association of Gerontology Conference: The age of celebration and expectation, Sydney, September 1999.

56 Mills N. The biomechanics of hip protectors. Proceedings of the Institution of Mechanical Engineers, Part H. *Journal of Engineering in Medicine* 1996;210:259–66.

57 Lauritzen JB, Petersen MM, Lund B. Effect of external hip protectors on hip fractures. *Lancet* 1993;341:11–13.

58 Wallace RB, Ross JE, Huston JC, Kundel C, Woodworth G. Iowa FICSIT trial: the feasibility of elderly wearing a hip joint protective garment to reduce hip fractures. *Journal of the American Geriatrics Society* 1993;41:338–40.

59 Ekman A, Mallmin H, Michaelsson K, Ljunghall S. External hip protectors to prevent osteoporotic hip fractures (letter). *Lancet* 1997;350:563–4.

60 Villar M, Hill P, Inskip H, Thompson P, Cooper C. Will elderly rest home residents wear hip protectors? *Age and Ageing* 1998;27:195–8.

61 Parkkari J, Heikkila J, Kannus P. Acceptability and compliance with wearing energy-shunting hip protectors: a 6-month prospective follow-up in a Finnish nursing home. *Age and Ageing* 1998;27:225–9.

62 Cameron I, Quine S. External hip protectors: likely non-compliance among high risk elderly people living in the community. *Archives of Gerontology and Geriatrics* 1994;19:273–81.

63 Birks C, Lockwood K, Cameron I, et al. Hip protectors: results of a user survey. *Australasian Journal on Ageing* 1999;18:23–6.

64 Cameron I, Kurrle S. External hip protectors (letter). *Journal of the American Geriatrics Society* 1997;45:1158.

65 Tinetti ME, Liu WL, Claus EB. Predictors and prognosis of inability to get up after falls among elderly persons. *Journal of the American Medical Association* 1993;269:65–70.

66 Reece AC, Simpson JM. Preparing older people to cope after a fall. *Physiotherapy* 1996;82:227–35.

67 Simpson JM, Harrington R, Marsh N. Guidelines for managing falls among elderly people. *Physiotherapy* 1998;84:173–7.

68 Tinetti M, Liu W-L, Marottoli R, Ginter S. Mechanical restraint use among residents of skilled nursing facilities. *Journal of the American Medical Association* 1991;265:468–71.

69 Watson ME, Mayhew PA. Identifying fall risk factors in preparation for reducing the use of restraints. *MEDSURG Nursing* 1994;3:25–8.

70 Capezuti E, Evans L, Strumpf N, Maislin G. Physical restraint use and falls in nursing home residents. *Journal of the American Geriatrics Society* 1996;44:627–33.

71 Rubenstein LZ, Josephson KR, Osterweil D. Falls and fall prevention in the nursing home. *Clinics in Geriatric Medicine* 1996;12:881–902.

72 Capezuti E, Strumpf N, Evans L, Grisso J, Maislin G. The relationship between physical restraint removal and falls and injuries among nursing home residents. *Journals of Gerontology: Series A, Biological and Medical Sciences* 1998;53:M47–52.

73 Werner P, Cohen-Mansfield J, Koroknay V, Braun J. The impact of a restraint-reduction programme on nursing home residents. *Geriatric Nursing* 1994;15:142–6.

74 Levine JM, Marchello V, Totolos E. Progress toward a restraint-free environment in a large academic nursing facility. *Journal of the American Geriatrics Society* 1995;43:914–18.

75 Ejaz FK, Folmar SJ, Kaufmann M, Rose MS, Goldman B: Restraint reduction: can it be achieved? *Gerontologist* 1994;34:694–9.

12

Prevention of falls in hospitals and residential aged care facilities

Many of the risk factors and prevention strategies outlined in previous sections are also relevant to falls among hospital patients and residents of hostels and nursing homes. However, a number of aspects are unique to institutional settings and the older people who reside within them. This chapter outlines risk factors for falling within hospitals and residential aged care facilities and an integrated approach to falls prevention in these settings.

Incidence and risk factors

Hospitals

Falls among patients are a key issue for hospitals. Up to a quarter of people fall during their time in a rehabilitation hospital [1] or ward [2]. These figures are even higher for particular diagnoses. For example, up to 40% of stroke patients fall while in a rehabilitation unit [3]. A number of risk factors for falls among hospital inpatients have been identified [1, 4–12] and are outlined in Table 12.1.

Several investigators have attempted to determine the relative importance of the various risk factors. In a case–control study involving 44 patients who fell during their acute hospital stays and 44 nonfallers (matched for sex, patient type and primary diagnosis), Salgado et al. [6] found that four of these variables were able to correctly classify 80% of patients into faller and nonfaller groups. These key variables were: impaired orientation, psychoactive drug use, evidence of stroke and impaired performance on the 'get-up-and-go test', which involves standing up from a chair, walking 5 m, turning around and returning [13].

Oliver et al. [12] found a different but related set of key predictors in an initial case–control study of 232 hospital patients. From this study they developed the STRATIFY (St Thomas's risk assessment tool in falling elderly inpatients) which involves assessment of: (i) whether falls are the presenting complaint; (ii) transfer and mobility skills; (iii) whether patient was agitated; (iv) needed frequent toileting, or (v) was visually impaired. This tool was then trialled in two large cohort studies (of 1217 and 331 patients) and found to have high sensitivity (ability to cor-

Table 12.1. Risk factors for falls in hospital

Confusion

Impaired orientation

Agitation

Depression

Visual impairment

Mobility impairment

Incontinence/diarrhoea/frequent toileting

Require assistance to toilet

Psychoactive medication use

Falls as a presenting complaint/history of falls

Comorbidity

Evidence of stroke

Primary cancer diagnosis

Congestive heart failure

Dizziness/vertigo

rectly identify people as fallers) and a good specificity (ability to correctly identify people as nonfallers). These findings indicate that simple, quick to administer assessment items are useful in identifying older persons at risk of falling while in hospital.

Residential aged care facilities

Falls incidence rates are as much as three times higher among older people in residential aged care settings than among community-dwelling older people [14]. This equates to an average annual rate of 1.5 falls per nursing home bed [14].

In a comprehensive prospective study involving 18 855 residents of 272 nursing homes, Kiely et al. [15] found that the most important predictor was a history of falls. Residents with a fall history were three times more likely to fall during the follow-up period than residents without such a history. Other independent risk factors were: wandering behaviour, use of a cane or walker, deterioration in activities of daily living performance, age greater than 87 years, unsteady gait, independence in performing transfers, not requiring a wheelchair and male gender. Interestingly, falling rates varied greatly among the nursing homes studied, and this was independent of patient-specific factors. This indicates the importance of broader design and management issues in falls prevention in residential aged care.

Risk factors for falling among nursing home residents have generally been found to be similar to those for community dwellers [16–18]. The increased prevalence of a number of important falls risk factors among people within institutional settings undoubtedly contributes to the greater incidence in this population. These are likely to include: muscle weakness, gait and balance disorders and dizziness or vertigo [14, 19], poor vision and dementia [20]. In addition, the increased prevalence of incontinence and antipsychotic drug use within institutions probably means that these factors are of greater relative importance in these settings.

An integrated approach to falls prevention in institutional settings

To prevent falls in hospital, hostel and nursing home settings, an integrated multifaceted approach is likely to offer the best chance of success. Such an approach should involve systems for identifying those at a high risk of falling, the implementation of strategies to minimize this risk, ongoing monitoring of falls rates and education of staff, patients and visitors about falls prevention [4, 21–24]. Components of such an approach are outlined in Table 12.2 and discussed below. More details on environmental risk factor modification, medical management and medications are given in Chapters 9, 13 and 14.

Screening protocols

Many hospitals use falls risk assessment tools to identify those at high risk of falling. For a screening tool to be useful, it must be quick and easy to administer and have a proven ability to identify likely fallers. The tools developed by Salgado et al. [6] and Oliver et al. [12] appear useful in this regard, although additional risk factors including orthostatic hypotension and other factors listed in Table 12.1 may also need to be considered for individual patients.

Within residential aged care facilities, more extensive screening for falls risk is possible as the residents are there for longer periods of time than hospital inpatients. A useful screening tool has been developed by the Centre for Education and Research on Ageing [24]. Assessment methods and management options are outlined for the following categories: medications, acute illness, mental state, ongoing medical conditions, history of falls, poor balance, use of walking aids, bowel or bladder problems, visual problems, hearing problems, foot problems and footwear. Of course other physiological risk factors (such as reduced muscle strength) outlined in Part I of this book will also be important and should be assessed.

Risk factor modification

Where possible, risk factors such as confusion, agitation, comorbidity, psychoactive medication use, adverse drug interactions, reduced muscle strength and poor balance, and poor vision should be investigated and addressed. This will need to be done in conjunction with the patient's medical practitioner and may also involve physiotherapy intervention and/or supervised exercise. Regular group exercise

Table 12.2. An integrated approach for preventing falls and falls injury

Use a screening protocol to identify high-risk patients

Address the risk factors directly if possible
Provide treatment of medical conditions that give rise to acute confusional states
Provide treatment/therapy for agitation
Provide treatment for comorbidity where possible
Monitor and attempt to remove or reduce dose of psychoactive drugs
Initiate online prescribing system to prevent adverse drug interactions
Initiate physiotherapy programmes that include specific muscle strengthening exercises, gait
   and balance training
Provide general exercise opportunities to prevent deterioration in motor function
Provide suitable walking aids
Ensure safe shoes and clothing are worn
Maximize vision with appropriate spectacles
Provide occupational therapy training programmes to maximize safety and independence in
   functional tasks
Ensure regular monitoring of patients/residents
Ensure regular assistance with toileting
Provide regular supervised walking for those unsafe to walk independently

Implement environmental interventions
Provide optimal lighting
Remove or modify obstacle hazards
Remove any hazardous floor covering
Bevel thresholds
Ensure regular maintenance of wheelchairs and other equipment
Minimize water and other spills on floors
Install grab rails in bathroom and toilet areas
Ensure toilet seats are of appropriate height
Provide appropriate height chairs
Provide easy access to call bells, light switches and personal effects
Provide toileting aids (urine bottles/bedside commodes/bedpans)
Provide other equipment (long-handle reachers, etc.)
Locate at-risk patients near nursing stations
Locate at-risk patients near bathrooms and dining rooms
Consider installation of electronic surveillance system
Provide safe walking areas for those who 'wander'
Consider use of restraints

Increase awareness of falls risk
Inform patients of their increased risk
Inform relatives of the patient's increased risk

Table 12.2. (*cont.*)

Consider method of quick identification of high-risk patients, e.g. coloured bracelet, code on
   patient file
Initiate and repeat educational programmes for staff
Ensure high level of monitoring during early days of hospital stay (staff/relatives)

Reduce falls injury
Implement hip protector programme for very high-risk patients (e.g. those with delirium,
   agitation, confusion and multiple risk factors)
Consider shock-absorbing floor surfaces
Consider low-height beds

Discharge planning
Undertake full assessment of functional abilities prior to discharge
Arrange appropriate assistance from carers and community services
Arrange for ongoing physiotherapy, community exercise, home assessment and modification
   and aged care team involvement as appropriate

Post-fall assessment
Document circumstances and investigate causes for each fall and intervene as appropriate
   Review environmental factors
   Review physical factors
   Perform functional assessment

opportunities such as exercise classes may also help prevent deterioration in motor
functioning, and supervised regular walking may be beneficial for unsafe walkers.
Occupational therapy training programmes may also be useful in maximizing safe
independence in functional tasks. There is evidence from one randomized controlled trial that more intensive physiotherapy and occupational therapy intervention for those in nursing homes leads to improved functional abilities (and a
resultant saving of nursing staff time) [25].

   It is also crucial that patients and residents be regularly monitored to ascertain if
they require assistance. In addition, those who are unable to toilet independently,
or are using laxatives or diuretics, may benefit from assistance with toileting at
regular intervals.

Environmental interventions

   Within hospitals and long-term care institutions, there should be the potential to
minimize environmental hazards. This would involve adequate monitoring and
maintenance of lighting, furniture, aids, equipment and floors. Transient environ-

mental hazards such as obstacles, clutter and spills on floors should also be quickly identified and rectified.

Attention should also be given to the way in which each individual patient or resident interacts with the environment. For example, a person with limited mobility needs to have easy access to personal effects (tissues, books, drinks) so they do not attempt to get up to fetch them, or reach for them in an unsafe manner. Similarly, a call bell should always be in easy reach of the person. This enables patients to call for assistance for completing daily tasks, and to alert staff quickly if they get into any difficulties. For those who are not able to move around their room independently yet have the cognitive and physical abilities to carry out some self-care tasks, toilet aids should be located within easy reach (e.g. urine bottles for men, bedpans or bedside commodes for women). In this way independence can be safely enhanced. Chairs should be height-adjustable so they can be set at a height from which it is easy for the person to stand up, as it is more difficult to stand up from a lower chair due to the extra muscle force required [26]. Those who can carry out daily tasks independently may benefit from an occupational therapy assessment and the provision of additional equipment, such as long-handled reachers for picking dropped objects up off the floor.

Safety can be maximized with careful consideration of the optimal location for individual patients/residents. For example, those with difficulty walking may benefit from being closer to bathrooms and dining rooms, while those at very high risk of falling should be located closer to staff stations where regular supervision is more possible.

The installation of electronic surveillance systems should also be considered to assist in monitoring high risk people. Such a system may involve video cameras, position sensors on beds or chairs or on an individual's lower limbs (to alert staff when a potential faller gets up) [27] or an alarm which is triggered when a person goes beyond a certain point.

While a number of the above strategies prevent older people moving unsafely, care must be taken that people are not unnecessarily restricted from standing up and walking, as this will contribute to greater losses of strength, balance and function, which in turn can lead to an increased risk of falls. Instead, regular supervised walking and exercise programmes should be undertaken. For those who 'wander', pleasant but safe walking areas should be provided.

Among those at very high risk of falling the use of restraints may be considered. The issue of restraints in institutional settings is a complicated and controversial one and is discussed in Chapter 11.

Increase awareness of falls risk

Education is a crucial part of any falls prevention programme [24]. Where appropriate, patients and residents should be informed of their increased risk of falls and the particular activities that they should avoid attempting unassisted or unsupervised. Similarly, relatives and other visitors and all staff who will come into contact with the patient or resident (including cleaners, food service staff, etc.) should also be apprised of this information. Systems are required to ensure that specific patient information is conveyed from each nursing shift to the next, and that no lapses in vigilance occur during staff changeovers [14]. Education sessions should also be held regularly due to staff and resident changes.

Reduce falls injury

Even the most conscientious application of a falls prevention programme will not totally eradicate falls, particularly among very high-risk individuals. Therefore, some attention must also be given to the prevention of injury following a fall. Strategies to consider include the provision of hip protectors (see Chapter 11 for details), shock-absorbing floor surfaces and low-height beds or mattresses on the floor to lessen the distance a patient or resident can fall.

Discharge planning

Programmes to prevent falls among hospital inpatients should not cease as soon as the person leaves the hospital. Effective discharge planning has a role to play in minimizing the risk of falls soon after return home. This is vital as several studies have shown that people recently discharged from hospital are at increased risk of falling. For example, Forster and Young [28] found that 73% of stroke patients fell in the 6 months after discharge from hospital. Similarly, Mahoney et al. [29] found that 14% of 214 older patients fell in the first month after returning home from a period of hospitalization for a medical illness.

Assessments of a person's functional abilities and risk of falling should be carried out prior to discharge from hospital. The person should not leave the hospital until it is clear that they are able safely to manage essential self-care and household tasks or assistance with these tasks has been arranged. This is especially important if an older person has spent a prolonged period of time in bed and is thus likely to be weaker than prior to the illness. An occupational therapy home visit may be necessary to establish safety at home, and has been shown to reduce falls rate among past fallers who have recently been in hospital [30]. Short periods of intensive rehabilitation should be considered for those recovering from major illness or surgery. Such a rehabilitation programme would aim to maximize the person's physical ability and thus independence.

Post-fall assessment

Is it vital that systems be put in place for the investigation of all falls that do occur [14]. Any environmental hazards associated with the fall should be identified and acted on as appropriate. A physical examination of the faller is important for the identification of any individual causes and risk factors. A review of the person's functional abilities and the interaction between these and the environment will also assist in identification of modifiable risk factors.

Evaluation of strategies for falls prevention in institutions

A recent trial has shown the efficacy of a falls prevention programme in nursing homes [31]. This study involved 482 residents who had previously fallen. Seven pairs of nursing homes were randomized to receive no intervention, or the intervention programme which involved structured individual assessment (of environmental safety, wheelchair use, psychotropic drug use and transfers and ambulation) by medical, nursing and occupational therapy professionals. At post-test there was a mean reduction of 19% in the proportion of recurrent fallers in the intervention homes. Greater effects were evident for homes with a higher compliance with recommendations and for residents with three or more previous falls. However, in a randomized controlled trial of a comprehensive post-fall assessment, Rubenstein et al. [32] found that while this approach reduced hospitalizations and hospital stays, it did not significantly reduce the rate of subsequent falls.

Only a few studies have investigated the effectiveness of falls prevention strategies in hospitals. Tideiksaar et al. [33] trialled a bed alarm system in a randomized controlled trial among 70 patients at high risk of falling. The device involved a sensor strip under the bedclothes which alerted nursing staff to a patient's attempt to get out of bed, thus enabling them to provide assistance. Although not statistically different, fewer falls occurred in the intervention group. Another study using historical controls [27] reports a decreased falls incidence following the introduction of a thigh position monitoring alarm. This device alerts staff when a person attempts to get out of bed or stand up. However, in a randomized controlled trial, Mayo et al. [34] found that an identification bracelet worn by those identified as being at high risk of falling was not effective in preventing falls.

Conclusion

Many older people within hospitals and aged care facilities are at increased risk of falling. There is now good evidence that a multidisciplinary, multifactorial assessment and intervention programme can be effective in reducing the risk of falls in nursing homes. Preliminary findings also indicate that patient movement alarms can prevent falls in hospital patients. While many of the strategies for preventing falls outlined above make good common sense, most have not been rigorously tested for their effectiveness and cost-effectiveness in research trials. The implemention of these strategies in institutional settings, therefore, requires further evaluation.

REFERENCES

1 Mayo NE, Korner-Bitensky N, Becker R, Georges P. Predicting falls among patients in a rehabilitation hospital. *American Journal of Physical Medicine and Rehabilitation* 1989;68:139–46.

2 Dromerick A, Reding M. Medical and neurological complications during inpatient stroke rehabilitation. *Stroke* 1994;25:358–61.

3 Nyberg L, Gustafson Y. Patient falls in stroke rehabilitation. A challenge to rehabilitation strategies. *Stroke* 1995;26:838–42.

4 Schmid NA. Reducing patient falls: a research-based comprehensive fall prevention programme. *Military Medicine* 1990;155:202–7.

5 Rapport LJ, Webster JS, Flemming KL, et al. Predictors of falls among right-hemisphere stroke patients in the rehabilitation setting. *Archives of Physical Medicine and Rehabilitation* 1993;74:621–6.

6 Salgado R, Lord SR, Packer J, Ehrlich F. Factors associated with falling in elderly hospital patients. *Gerontology* 1994;40:325–31.

7 Bates DW, Pruess K, Souney P, Platt R. Serious falls in hospitalized patients: correlates and resource utilization. *American Journal of Medicine* 1995;99:137–43.

8 Gales BJ, Menard SM: Relationship between the administration of selected medications and falls in hospitalized elderly patients. *Annals of Pharmacotherapy* 1995;29:354–8.

9 Hendrich A, Nyhuis A, Kippenbrock T, Soja ME. Hospital falls: development of a predictive model for clinical practice. *Applied Nursing Research* 1995;8:129–39.

10 Gluck T, Wientjes HJ, Rai GS. An evaluation of risk factors for in-patient falls in acute and rehabilitation elderly care wards. *Gerontology* 1996;42:104–7.

11 Nyberg L, Gustafson Y. Fall prediction index for patients in stroke rehabilitation. *Stroke* 1997;28:716–21.

12 Oliver D, Britton M, Seed P, Martin FC, Hopper AH. Development and evaluation of evidence-based risk assessment tool (STRATIFY) to predict which elderly inpatients will fall: case–control and cohort studies. *British Medical Journal* 1997;315:1049–53.

13 Mathias S, Nayak US, Isaacs B. Balance in elderly patients: the 'get-up and go' test. *Archives of Physical Medicine & Rehabilitation* 1986;67:387–9.

14 Rubenstein LZ, Josephson KR, Osterweil D. Falls and fall prevention in the nursing home. *Clinics in Geriatric Medicine* 1996;12:881–902.

15 Kiely DK, Kiel DP, Burrows AB, Lipsitz LA. Identifying nursing home residents at risk for falling. *Journal of the American Geriatrics Society* 1998;46:551–5.

16 Lipsitz LA, Jonsson PV, Kelley MM, Koestner JS. Causes and correlates of recurrent falls in ambulatory frail elderly. *Journal of Gerontology* 1991;46:M114–22.

17 Luukinen H, Koski K, Laippala P, Kivela SL. Risk factors for recurrent falls in the elderly in long-term institutional care. *Public Health* 1995;109:57–65.

18 Thapa PB, Gideon P, Fought RL, Ray WA. Psychotropic drugs and risk of recurrent falls in ambulatory nursing home residents. *American Journal of Epidemiology* 1995;142:202–11.

19 Rubenstein LZ, Josephson KR, Robbins AS. Falls in the nursing home. *Annals of Internal Medicine* 1994;121:442–51.

20 Jantti PO, Pyykko VI, Hervonen AL. Falls among elderly nursing home residents. *Public Health* 1993;107:89–96.

21 Hendrich A. An effective unit-based fall prevention plan. *Journal of Nursing Quality Assurance* 1988;3:28–36.

22 Foster KS, Kohlenberg EM. Patient falls in a tertiary rehabilitation setting. *Rehabilitation Nursing Research* 1996;5:23–9.

23 Joanna Briggs Institute for Evidence-Based Nursing: Falls in hospitals: best practice: *Evidence-based information sheets for health professionals* 1998;2:1–6.

24 Shanley C. *Putting your best foot forward: preventing and managing falls in aged care facilities.* Sydney: The Centre for Education and Research on Ageing (CERA), 1998.

25 Przybylski B, Dumont E, Watkins M, Warren S, Beaulne A, Lier D. Outcomes of enhanced physical and occupational therapy service in a nursing home setting. *Archives of Physical Medicine and Rehabilitation* 1996;77:554–61.

26 Arborelius U, Wretenberg P, Lindberg F. The effects of armrests and high seat heights on lower-limb joint load and muscular activity during sitting and rising. *Ergonomics* 1992;35:1377–91.

27 Widder B. A new device to decrease falls. *Geriatric Nursing: American Journal of Care for the Aging* 1985;6:287–8.

28 Forster A, Young J. Incidence and consequences of falls due to stroke: a systematic inquiry. *British Medical Journal* 1995;311:83–6.

29 Mahoney J, Sager M, Dunham NC, Johnson J. Risk of falls after hospital discharge. *Journal of the American Geriatrics Society* 1994;42:269–74.

30 Cumming R, Thomas M, Szonyi G, et al. Home visits by an occupational therapist for assessment and modification of environmental hazards: a randomized controlled trial of falls prevention. *Journal of the American Geriatrics Society* 1999;47:1397–1402.

31 Ray WA, Taylor JA, Meador KG, et al. A randomized trial of a consultation service to reduce falls in nursing homes. *Journal of the American Medical Association* 1997;278:557–62.

32 Rubenstein LZ, Robbins AS, Josephson KR, Schulman BL, Osterweil D. The value of assessing falls in an elderly population. A randomized clinical trial. *Annals of Internal Medicine* 1990;113:308–16.

33 Tideiksaar R, Feiner CF, Maby J. Falls prevention: the efficacy of a bed alarm system in an acute-care setting. *Mount Sinai Journal of Medicine* 1993;60:522–7.

34 Mayo NE, Gloutney L, Levy AR. A randomized trial of identification bracelets to prevent falls among patients in a rehabilitation hospital. *Archives of Physical Medicine & Rehabilitation* 1994;75:1302–8.

13

The medical management of older people at risk of falls

As indicated in Part I of this book there are many intrinsic risk factors for falls in older people. It is apparent that some can not be modified, whereas others may respond to a range of treatments. Regardless of whether each measure is amenable to modification, appropriate management is required, and general practitioners need to be equipped to carry out this task. This chapter addresses the implications of the research findings presented in Chapters 4, 5 and 7, and presents guidelines for an informed approach to the medical management of older persons at risk of falling. It also recommends simple tests for vision, sensation, strength, reaction time and balance that could be performed in general practice settings to complement a routine medical assessment.

Medical management of conditions associated with falls

As outlined in Chapters 4, 5 and 7, many medical conditions and medications have been found to be risk factors for falls in community and institutional settings. In particular, cognitive impairment, stroke, Parkinson's disease, and use of psychoactive medications have consistently been found to increase falls risk. However, many other medical conditions (such as orthostatic hypotension, foot problems and vestibular pathology) which have not have been found to be strong risk factors in large population studies, may be of considerable importance to individuals. Therefore, the general practitioner plays an important role in both the diagnosis and management of these conditions in older people.

The medical management of older people at risk of falls often involves a multidisciplinary approach, which requires good communication between the practitioner, the patient, other health professionals involved in the older person's medical care, and family or carers in the patient's home environment. In Table 13.1, we have outlined suggestions for the management of the medical risk factors considered in Chapters 4, 5 and 7. The table also provides suggestions for appropriate referral.

Table 13.1. Suggestions for management of medical risk factors in general practice

Risk factor	GP management	Referral/liaison
Eye disease (inc. age-related maculopathy, cataracts, glaucoma)	Routine eye examination, repeat prescriptions of topical eye medications, education	Ophthalmologist, optometrist, occupational therapist
Foot disorders (inc. corns and calluses, bunions, nail problems, ulceration)	Scalpel reduction of calluses, orthotic devices/insoles, footwear and home footcare advice and education	Podiatrist, orthopaedic surgeon, orthotist, boot-maker
Musculoskeletal disorders (inc. osteoarthritis, rheumatoid arthritis, acute soft tissue injuries)	Appropriate diagnostic evaluation, anti-inflammatory drugs, mobility aids (frames, walking sticks) self-treatment education, prescription of hip protectors, exercise advice	Physiotherapist, orthopaedic surgeon, prosthetist, orthotist, rheumatologist, occupational therapist
Peripheral neuropathy	Manage diabetes, screen for vitamin B_{12} deficiency, walking stick, education regarding improving walking safety, foot orthoses	Neurologist, endocrinologist, physiotherapist, podiatrist
Use of medications	Minimise total medications taken, assess risk and benefits of each medication, prescribe lowest effective dose, frequent reassessment, education	Pharmacist, geriatrician, aged care facility staff
Orthostatic hypotension	Assessment of medications, rehydration	Cardiologist, aged care facility staff
Vestibular dysfunction	Avoidance of drugs with vestibular effects, otolaryngological evaluation	Otolaryngologist, neurologist
Neurological disorders (inc. stroke, cerebellar disorders, Parkinson's disease)	Appropriate diagnostic evaluation, prescription of hip protectors	Neurologist, geriatrician, physiotherapist, occupational therapist
Psychological factors (inc. dementia, depression, anxiety, delerium)	Detect reversible causes, take care with prescription of centrally acting drugs, prescription of hip protectors	Neurologist, psychiatrist, psychologist, aged care facility staff

Table 13.1. (*cont.*)

Risk factor	GP management	Referral/liaison
Incontinence	Appropriate diagnostic evaluation, advice, assessment of diuretic use	Urologist, continence nurse, gynaecologist, physiotherapist, occupational therapist, aged care facility staff
Severe and recurrent dizziness	Appropriate diagnostic evaluation to determine cause	Otolaryngologist, neurologist, cardiologist

Counselling the older adult at risk of falling

One of the most important roles for a general practitioner when managing an older patient at risk of falling is to provide practical advice relating to the specific impairments revealed by their clinical assessments. This assists the older patient in playing an active role in minimizing the risks generated by their sensorimotor deficits. In Figures 13.1–13.3, we have provided a list of practical suggestions for general practitioners to pass on to older patients with impaired strength, balance and coordination, peripheral sensory loss, and impaired vision. A footwear advice handout is also provided, based on the research findings discussed in Chapter 10 (see Figure 13.4).

General practice assessment of the at-risk older patient

General practitioners are subject to many competing demands on their time, which results in time spent with each individual patient being necessarily brief. Therefore, a rapid falls assessment tool is required to assist in identifying causative factors in people at risk of falls. However, as indicated in Chapter 4, the utility of a falls risk assessment based solely on diagnoses of disease processes is of questionable value. Furthermore, the predictive value of some standard clinical tests such as high-contrast eye charts for assessing vision, tuning forks for measuring vibration sense, strength using the five-point grading scale and the Rhomberg balance test is also limited.

To address these issues, we have devised a brief assessment suitable for general practice, based on the sensorimotor functional model for falls prediction developed by our research group. Although many other tests have been suggested as 'single' falls predictors (such as the functional reach test [1]), we feel that a sensorimotor model is preferable as it allows the general practitioner to not only predict which older patients are likely to fall, but also to determine which sensorimotor systems are impaired. This gives greater insight into the causes of instability and

---

INFORMATION ON HOW TO IMPROVE STRENGTH, COORDINATION AND BALANCE

How can these factors lead to falls ?
Adequate strength is required to support the body weight as we stand and walk. A weakness in one leg can result in a fall when all of the body weight is placed on it. Strength is also important for undertaking every day activities such as getting out of bed, rising from a chair and walking up and down steps.

Good static and dynamic balance are required so we keep control of our upright bodies and quick reaction time and good coordination allow us to recover in time if we trip, stumble or lose balance.

What you can do

▪ the best treatment for any reduced functioning in the above factors is exercise.

▪ exercise classes designed for older people are particularly beneficial, as any specific balance, strength or coordination problem can be targeted. Exercising in a group also provides a structure and social support.

▪ specific home exercises and increased general exercise such as walking, gardening etc. provide important additional benefits.

Fig. 13.1.   Patient information regarding strength, coordination and balance.

falls and provides guidance for the type/s of intervention that will most benefit the patient.

The sensitivity of this battery of tests is inevitably lower than that which could be expected from more detailed quantitative assessments – as described in Chapter 16. However, poor performances in each of the assessment items will enable the identification of 'high risk' fallers in the context of general practice. The falls assessment includes functional measures of the major physiological systems that contribute to standing balance and is designed to complement the systematic management of medical conditions as outlined in Table 13.1. It requires minimal equipment: a low contrast eye chart, an aesthesiometer filament for measuring touch sensation and a calibrated wooden rod for measuring reaction time (this equipment and testing instructions can be obtained from the authors), in addition to a sphygmomanometer for measuring blood pressure changes. At present we are evaluating the predictive value of these assessments, the feasibility and utility of this approach in general practice.

INFORMATION ON HOW TO COMPENSATE FOR SENSATION LOSS

How can sensation loss lead to falls?
Leg sensation provides information to the brain about your standing position and your leg movements as you undertake activities like walking and getting in and out of a chair. Imagine if your legs were totally numb – they would provide no information to the brain at all.

What you can do

- take particular care when walking on surfaces that are uneven or soft, i.e. footpaths, uneven or rough ground and thick carpets and rugs.
- avoid walking in dim or unlit areas if possible and make sure you turn the light on before walking in the house at night.
- wear shoes with low heels and firm rubber soles to maximise leg sensation and balance.
- consider using a walking stick or light cane as a sensor (rather than/or in addition to a support) to help you compensate for sensation loss. For example a stick gives extra information about footpath and road cracks and irregularities.

Fig. 13.2.   Patient information regarding sensory loss.

Figure 13.5 presents the falls risk assessment checklist. This one-page form provides the criterion values for poor performances in the tests and spaces for indicating action taken and a review date.

Vision

Vision is usually assessed in primary care setting using high-contrast letter charts (Snellen scales) or cruder assessments, such as testing ability to read printed material. These tests are not optimal for measuring visual requirements for detecting environment hazards, particularly under suboptimal conditions such as when contrast is reduced. A more appropriate test for measuring whether poor vision may predispose an older person to fall is an assessment of low contrast visual acuity [2] (see Figure 13.6). For example, we have found that poor low-contrast visual acuity is a better predictor of falls than high-contrast visual acuity in both institutionalized [3] and community-dwelling [4] people. Low-contrast visual acuity is tested in a standard manner, that is by asking patients to read the smallest line of

---

INFORMATION ON HOW TO MAXIMISE VISION

How can reduced vision lead to falls?
People with reduced vision have an increased risk of tripping over objects within the home and especially when outside in unfamiliar surroundings. This is particularly the case in circumstances that are sub-optimal, e.g. in poor lighting conditions, at dusk, in high glare situations and when the light intensity changes – i.e. going from bright light into the dark and vice versa.

Bifocals, trifocals and multifocals make things worse - even in those who have been wearing them for years. The problem with these glasses is that their lower sections blur obstacles on the ground we need to see to avoid tripping.

What you can do

- have your eyes assessed every year by an eye doctor.
- wear only a single-lens pair of glasses (i.e. no bifocals, trifocals or multifocals) when walking, especially when outside the home.
- wear your glasses; don't keep them in a drawer or in your pocket.
- wear a hat and/or sunglasses when outside, especially in bright and high glare situations.
- avoid dimly lit areas if possible and turn the light on before walking in the house at night.
- put on your glasses if you get up in the night to go to the toilet.

Fig. 13.3.   Patient information regarding maximizing vision.

letters on the chart they can see from a set distance (usually 3 m). A Snellen fraction score of greater than 6/20 indicates significantly impaired low-contrast visual acuity.

Sensation

As outlined in Chapter 3, the ageing process is associated with impaired performance in tests of tactile sensitivity, vibration sense, and proprioception. Age-related peripheral sensory loss is a major risk factor for falls [5–7], and therefore, a thorough evaluation of an older patient at risk of falling should include an assessment of peripheral sensation. There is a diverse array of instruments available for the assessment of sensory loss, including tuning forks [8], biothesiometers [9] and touch aesthesiometers [10]. Each has its own advantages and disadvantages, however we suggest that the simplest and most accurate instrument for the

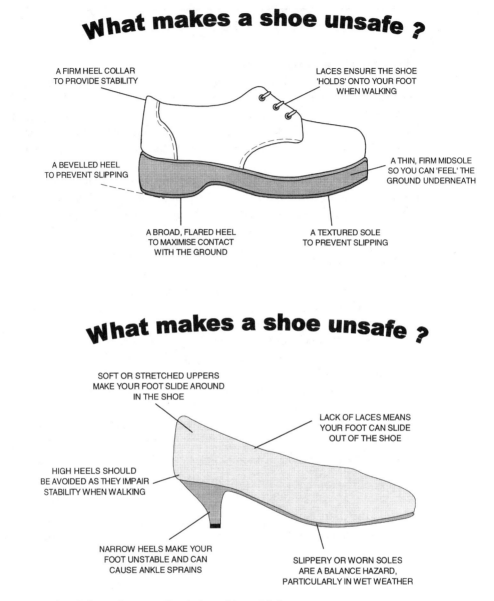

Fig. 13.4.   Patient information regarding 'safe and 'unsafe' shoes.

GENERAL PRACTICE FALLS RISK ASSESSMENT CHECKLIST

Dr:_____   Assessment date:_____

Patient:_____   Date of birth:_____

Address:_____   Phone:_____

ASSESSMENT	✓	ACTION TAKEN	REVIEW DATE
Vision[1] - low contrast visual acuity test > 6/20			
Sensation[2] - inability to detect 4.56 filament			
Strength[3] -unable to sit-to-stand from standard (45cm) height chair in ≤ 2 sec without arm support			
Reaction time[4] -rod catch measure > 300 milliseconds (best of three attempts)			
Balance[5] -requires step in 30sec near-tandem standing test (eyes closed)			

ACTION

1. Examine for glaucoma, cataracts, and suitability of eyewear. Refer to optometrist or ophthalmologist as necessary.
2. Manage diabetes, screen for vitamin B12 deficiency, counselling. Refer to neurologist, endocrinologist and physiotherapist as necessary.
3. Appropriate diagnostic evaluation. Encourage participation in local balance and strength improvement class and/or home exercises. Refer to physiotherapist or occupational therapist as necessary.
4. Screen for dementia, delerium, confusion and neurological conditions. Encourage participation in exercise classes and/or home exercises. Refer to neurologist as necessary.
5. Appropriate diagnostic evaluation. Encourage participation in local balance and strength improvement class and/or home exercises. Refer to neurologist or otolaryngologist as necessary.

Fig. 13.5.   Falls risk assessment checklist.

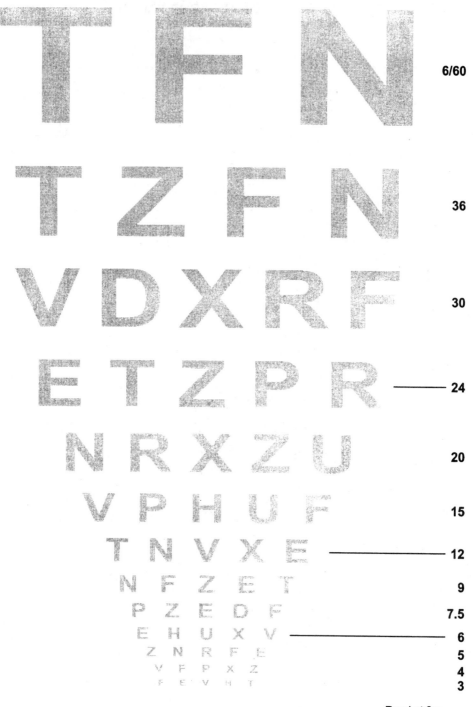

T F N — 6/60

T Z F N — 36

V D X R F — 30

E T Z P R — 24

N R X Z U — 20

V P H U F — 15

T N V X E — 12

N F Z E T — 9

P Z E D F — 7.5

E H U X V — 6

Z N R F E — 5

V F P X Z — 4

F E V H T — 3

Read at 3m

Fig. 13.6.   The low contrast visual acuity chart.

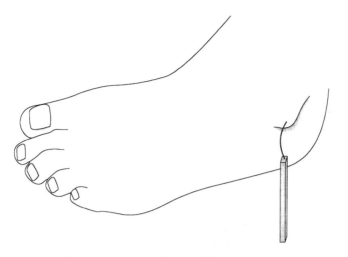

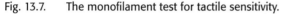

Fig. 13.7.   The monofilament test for tactile sensitivity.

screening of sensory loss in general practice is a single-monofilament aesthe-siometer (see Figure 13.7).

Sensory threshold testing with touch aesthesiometers has been found to be highly reliable [11], and correlates well with biopsy findings of peripheral nerve damage [12]. Peripheral sensory loss with ageing is most evident in the lower extremity [13–15], and many studies have reported that loss of sensation in the legs and feet is associated with impaired balance [16, 17] and increased risk of falling [5–7]. For these reasons, we suggest that tactile sensitivity should be assessed at the ankle (specifically, the lateral malleolus), as this site is a bony landmark that is easily palpable and provides a good indicator of lower limb sensation. An inability to detect the monofilament which exerts a pressure of 2.3 g represents significant peripheral sensory loss.

Strength

As outlined in Chapter 3, decreased lower limb muscle strength is associated with increased falls risk [18, 19]. Accordingly, assessment of muscle strength is an important component of a physiological test battery in clinical practice. However, the commonly employed five-point grading scale suffers from a severe ceiling effect and is not accurate enough to detect subtle but significant muscle weakness in older people. We suggest the 'sit-to-stand' functional strength test [20], as it is easy to administer and has been found to be a good predictor of falls [21–23] and deterioration in other aspects of daily functioning (Figure 13.8) [24, 25]. A stan-dard height chair (top of seat approximately 45 cm from the floor) is recommended as the amount of muscle force required to stand from the seated position varies

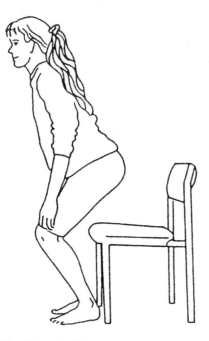

Fig. 13.8.   The sit-to-stand test.

with chair height [26]. To perform this test, the patient is seated in a chair, and then asked to stand up without using their arms for assistance. An inability to complete this task in 2 seconds indicates lower limb muscle weakness.

Reaction time

Reaction time declines with increasing age [27], and numerous studies have reported slow reaction time to be associated with an increased risk of falls [3, 28]. However, most tests of reaction time involve the use of specialized apparatus to provide the subject with an auditory or visual cue and a timing mechanism to measure accurately the period between the cue and the response. In the context of general practice, a simple alternative is a rod catch test, i.e. asking patients, while seated, to catch a wooden rod that is dropped vertically from just above the top of the hand (see Figure 13.9). By noting where the patient catches the rod (which is marked in milliseconds and indicates the time taken for the rod to fall under gravity), a measurement of reaction time can be obtained. Pilot investigations by our group have found that reaction times measured using this simple device are closely correlated (r=0.7) with finger-press reaction times requiring more specialized equipment. Failure to catch the rod within 300 milliseconds indicates significantly increased reaction time.

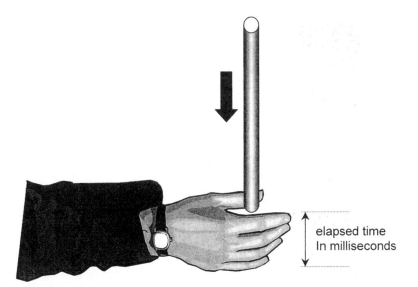

Fig. 13.9.   The 'rod catch test'. The point where the patient catches the rod is recorded as a measure of simple reaction time.

Balance

A wide range of balance tests have been described in the literature, however many require specialized equipment and are therefore not practical in the general practice environment. The sharpened Rhomberg test, in which the subject stands with one foot in front of the other (referred to as the 'tandem position"), has been widely recommended as a simple clinical measure of balance. However it is limited in that many older people are simply unable to perform the test, particularly with their eyes closed [29]. Similarly, the ability to stand on one leg has also been recommended as a simple measure of balance, but this is also difficult for older people to undertake [29, 30] and only moderately good at predicting falls [31, 32].

We have developed a new measure of standing balance which overcomes many of the shortcomings of the above tests, i.e. it is feasible for older people to undertake, yet discriminates between fallers and nonfallers [33]. This test requires patients to stand in a near-tandem position for 30 seconds with eyes closed, that is with the feet separated by 2.5 cm and the heel of the front foot 2.5 cm anterior to the toe of the back foot (Figure 13.10). An inability to hold the standing position without taking a protective step in the 30-second test period indicates poor balance.

The assessment of orthostatic hypotension

As discussed in Chapter 4, orthostatic hypotension has not been found to be a strong risk factor for falls in large population studies. However, as indicated in

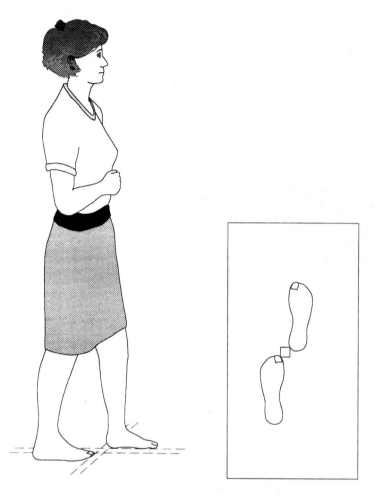

Fig. 13.10. The near-tandem standing balance test. The feet are separated by 2.5 cm and the heel of the front foot is positioned 2.5 cm anterior to the toe of the back foot.

Chapter 7, this may be due to study limitations including the sometimes-intermittent nature of this condition. As clinical experience indicates that orthostatic hypotension is a cause of falling in particular individuals, we suggest that an assessment of lying and standing blood pressure be included in a falls assessment for patients who suffer from unexplained falls and/or dizziness. Orthostatic hypotension is defined as a drop in systolic pressure of 20 mmHg or more, or diastolic pressure of 10 mmHg or more at 1–5 minutes after moving from the supine to the standing position. Patient reports of dizziness, lightheadedness and faintness during the procedure should also be noted.

Conclusion

Falls have a multifactorial aetiology, and therefore the medical management of older people at risk of falling requires a tailored approach for each individual. In this chapter, we have provided some suggestions for screening of older people at risk of falls based on our sensorimotor model, as this allows general practitioners to identify specific areas of concern. In addition, we have outlined some simple, practical approaches to managing medical conditions associated with falls, highlighting the importance of a multidisciplinary approach and the need to involve patients actively in reducing their falls risk.

REFERENCES

1 Duncan PW, Studenski S, Chandler J, Prescott B. Functional reach: predictive validity in a sample of elderly male veterans. *Journal of Gerontology* 1992;47(3):M93–8.
2 Verbaken JH, Johnston AW. Clinical contrast sensitivity testing; the current status. *Clinical and Experimental Optometry* 1986;69:204–12.
3 Lord SR, Clark RD, Webster IW. Physiological factors associated with falls in an elderly population. *Journal of the American Geriatrics Society* 1991;39:1194–200.
4 Lord SR, Sambrook PN, Gilbert C, et al. Postural stability, falls and fractures in the elderly: results from the Dubbo osteoporosis epidemiology study. *Medical Journal of Australia* 1994;160:684–5, 688–91.
5 Sorock GS, Labiner DM. Peripheral neuromuscular dysfunction and falls in an elderly cohort. *American Journal of Epidemiology* 1992;136:584–91.
6 Richardson JK, Hurvitz EA. Peripheral neuropathy: a true risk factor for falls. *Journal of Gerontology* 1995;50(4):M211–15.
7 Lord SR, Clark RD. Simple physiological and clinical tests for the accurate prediction of falling in older people. *Gerontology* 1996;42:199–203.
8 Thivolet C, ElFarkh J, Petiot A, Simonet C, Tourniaire J. Measuring vibration sensations with graduated tuning fork. *Diabetes Care* 1990;13:1077–80.
9 Bloom S, Till S, Sonksen P, Smith S. Use of a biothesiometer to measure individual vibration thresholds and their variation in 519 non-diabetic subjects. *British Medical Journal* 1984;288:1793–5.
10 Kumar S, Fernando DJS, Veves A, Knowles EA, Young MJ, Boulton AJM. Semmes–Weinstein monofilaments: a simple, effective and inexpensive screening device for identifying diabetic patients at risk of foot ulceration. *Diabetes Research and Clinical Practice* 1991;13:63–8.
11 Holewski JJ, Stess RM, Graf PM, Grunfeld C. Aesthesiometry: quantification of cutaneous pressure sensation in diabetic peripheral neuropathy. *Journal of Rehabilitation Research and Development* 1988;25:1–10.
12 Dyck PJ, O'Brien PC, Bushek W, Oviatt KF, Schilling K, Stevens JC. Clinical vs quantitative evaluation of cutaneous sensation. *Archives of Neurology* 1976;33:651–5.

13 Bolton CF, Winkelmann RK, Dyck PJ. A quantitative study of Meissner's corpuscles in man. *Neurology* 1966;16:1–9.

14 Dyck PJ, Schultz PW, O'Brien PC. Quantitation of touch-pressure sensation. *Archives of Neurology* 1972;26:465–73.

15 Kenshalo DR Sr. Somesthetic sensitivity in young and elderly humans. *Journal of Gerontology* 1986;41:732–42.

16 Lord SR, Clark RD, Webster IW. Postural stability and associated physiological factors in a population of aged persons. *Journal of Gerontology* 1991;46:M69–76.

17 Duncan G, Wilson JA, MacLennan WJ, Lewis S. Clinical correlates of sway in elderly people living at home. *Gerontology* 1992;38:160–6.

18 Lord SR, McLean D, Stathers G. Physiological factors associated with injurious falls in older people living in the community. *Gerontology* 1992;38:338–46.

19 Lord SR, Ward JA, Williams P, Anstey KJ. Physiological factors associated with falls in older community-dwelling women. *Journal of the American Geriatrics Society* 1994;42:1110–17.

20 Csuka M, McCarty DJ. Simple method for measurement of lower extremity muscle strength. *American Journal of Medicine* 1985;78:77–81.

21 Nevitt MC, Cummings SR, Kidd S, Black D. Risk factors for recurrent nonsyncopal falls. A prospective study. *Journal of the American Medical Association* 1989;261:2663–8.

22 Lipsitz LA, Jonsson PV, Kelley MM, Koestner JS. Causes and correlates of recurrent falls in ambulatory frail elderly. *Journal of Gerontology* 1991;46:M114–122.

23 Campbell AJ, Borrie MJ, Spears GF. Risk factors for falls in a community-based prospective study of people 70 years and older. *Journal of Gerontology* 1989;44:M112–17.

24 Guralnik J, Ferrucci L, Simonsick E, Salive M, Wallace R. Lower-extremity function in persons over the age of 70 years as a predictor of subsequent disability. *New England Journal of Medicine* 1995;332:556–61.

25 Gill TM, Williams CS, Tinetti ME. Assessing risk for the onset of functional dependence among older adults: the role of physical performance. *Journal of the American Geriatrics Society* 1995;43:603–9.

26 Arborelius U, Wretenberg P, Lindberg F. The effects of armrests and high seat heights on lower-limb joint load and muscular activity during sitting and rising. *Ergonomics* 1992;35:1377–91.

27 Welford AT. Motor performance. In: Birren JE, Schaie KW, editors. *Handbook of the Psychology of Aging.* New York: Van Nostrand Reinhold, 1997.

28 Grabiner MD, Jahnigen DW. Modeling recovery from stumbles: preliminary data on variable selection and classification efficacy. *Journal of the American Geriatrics Society* 1992;40:910–13.

29 Fregly AR, Smith MJ, Graybiel A. Revised normative standards of performance of men on a quantitative ataxia test battery. *Acta Otolaryngologica* 1973;75:10–16.

30 Crosbie WJ, Nimmo MA, Banks MA, Brownlee MG, Meldrum F. Standing balance responses in two populations of elderly women: a pilot study. *Archives of Physical Medicine & Rehabilitation* 1989;70:751–4.

31 Maki BE, Holliday PJ, Topper AK. A prospective study of postural balance and risk of falling in an ambulatory and independent elderly population. *Journal of Gerontology* 1994;49:M72–84.

32 Vellas BJ, Wayne SJ, Romero L, Baumgartner RN, Rubenstein LZ, Garry PJ. One-leg balance is an important predictor of injurious falls in older persons. *Journal of the American Geriatrics Society* 1997;45:735–8.

33 Lord SR, Rogers MW, Howland A, Fitzpatrick RC. Lateral stability, sensori-motor function and falls in older people. *Journal of the American Geriatrics Society* 1999;47:1077–81.

14

Modifying medication use to prevent falls

As outlined in Chapter 5, medication usage in older people is common, and certain classes of medications significantly increase risk of falling. In particular, psycho-active medications have been found to reduce mental alertness and impair balance in older people, and the use of these drugs is associated with an increased risk of falling. Furthermore, the use of multiple medications by older people increases the risk of adverse drug interactions [1], and is also associated with increased falls risk. In this chapter, we review the literature pertaining to medication withdrawal as a falls prevention strategy, and discuss the practical implications for modifying medication usage in older people. We also discuss alternatives to pharmacological treatment of anxiety, depression and sleep disturbances in older people.

Medication withdrawal and falls

Numerous strategies can be used to address medication use in older people, including minimizing the total number of drugs taken, assessing the risks and benefits of each drug, choosing drugs which are less centrally acting and do not produce postural hypotension, and reducing dose to the lowest possible effective level [2]. However, reducing medication use in older people is difficult, and prescribing habits are only partly influenced by the practitioner's knowledge of the risks associated with polypharmacy. Educational programmes regarding polypharmacy presented by pharmaceutical companies ('academic detailing') have not been found to be effective in reducing the total number of drugs prescribed to older people [3], although programmes directed at improving prescription of specific therapeutic classes have [4,5].

Involving the older person in the ongoing review of their medication use may be a useful strategy to minimize the risks associated with polypharmacy. Table 14.1 provides a list of simple guidelines for older people to become more aware of their medication use and prevent unnecessary duplication of drugs, and Figure 14.1 shows a simple medication record card which may assist in this process. However, a recent report suggests that medicine record cards will only be helpful if patients

Table 14.1. Simple guidelines for older people to become more aware of their medication use and prevent misuse of medications

Ask your doctor to review your medicines or ask your pharmacist for advice

Tell your doctor about any problems you are experiencing with your medication

Keep a record of which drugs you take by filling in a medication record card

Tell your doctor about any other doctors or specialists you may be seeing and any medicines they have prescribed

Take all your medications when you visit your doctor(s)

Do not use out of date medications

Do not use other people's medications

If you forget to take your medication, do not 'double-up' the next day

Ask your doctor if there are any nondrug alternatives to the management of your condition

MEDICATION RECORD CARD				
DATE PRESCRIBED	MEDICINE NAME AND STRENGTH	WHAT IT IS FOR	HOW MANY AND HOW OFTEN	OTHER INSTRUCTIONS

Fig. 14.1.   A medication record card for use by older people.

believe that their doctors want them to use such a device, as some doctors confess that they perceive medication cards as additional paperwork for each consultation and find them irritating rather than beneficial [6].

Withdrawal of medications is not easy, and in itself may produce detrimental effects if performed too quickly. For example, rapid withdrawal of psychoactive medications may lead to confusion and restlessness [7], which may impair an older person's ability to navigate obstacles in their environment [8]. Nevertheless, the benefits of appropriate withdrawal of psychoactive medication are significant, and may not necessarily be associated with increased psychological problems [9].

The ideal design for exploring the association between medication use and falls and/or falls injuries is a large controlled randomized trial wherein falls are prospectively measured [10,11]. In recent years, a few such studies have been performed. These studies have either focused on modifying the use of a single drug class such as the psychoactive or antihypertensives or have included drug use modification as a significant part of a multifaceted intervention [12,13].

In a randomized controlled trial of gradual psychoactive medication withdrawal and home-based exercise, Campbell et al. [13] found a significant reduction in falls in the older community-dwelling women randomized to the medication withdrawal arms of the study. This is a very encouraging finding as the risk of falling for those who completed the trial was reduced by 65%. However, there were considerable problems encountered in undertaking this study, which emphasizes how difficult it is for older people to stop using psychoactive medications. First, it proved very difficult to recruit subjects into the trial, with 400 of the 493 (81%) eligible subjects declining participation. Further, of the 48 subjects who agreed to participate and were randomized to the psychoactive withdrawal programmes, only 17 (35%) completed the trial. Eight of the 17 subjects who successfully completed the trial also restarted taking psychoactive medications within 1 month of the completion of the study.

Particularly in recognition of the problems associated with polypharmacy, a number of intervention studies have also been performed to reduce medication usage in nursing home residents [9, 14, 15], and there is a general consensus that reducing the use of psychoactive medications should be a major priority of physicians, pharmacists and nursing staff [10]. Rubenstein et al. [16] reported that a multiple intervention approach involving exercise, environmental modifications and altering drug intake did not produce a significantly reduced prevalence of falls in 160 residential care subjects. However, more recently Ray et al. [17] conducted a study involving 482 residents who had previously fallen in seven pairs of nursing homes. The nursing homes were randomized to receive an intervention programme which involved review of psychoactive drug use as well as interventions to improve transfers and ambulation, wheelchair use and environmental safety. They found that the proportion of recurrent fallers in the intervention homes decreased significantly (by 19%). At least part of this reduction in falls appears to have been due to the reduction in psychoactive medication use in the intervention nursing homes.

The available literature would therefore suggest that reducing psychoactive medication use to lower risk of falling is justified. However, evidence of potential benefits of reducing other medications is not so clear. Reduction in NSAID use to prevent falls has been questioned, as this may lead to an increase in arthritic pain and associated reduction in walking speed and general mobility [18, 19]. However, prescription of exercise may be able to compensate for NSAID withdrawal. The risks involved with withdrawing antihypertensive medications would appear to far outweigh the potential benefits of falls risk reduction [20], and as such, this approach is not generally regarded as a practical falls prevention strategy. Nonetheless, ongoing monitoring of blood pressure should be undertaken to maintain optimal antihypertensive dosage.

Alternatives to pharmacological treatments of anxiety, depression and sleep disturbances in older people

Due to the increased risk of falls and other significant adverse side effects of psycho-active medications in older people, alternative nonpharmacological therapies for the treatment of anxiety, depression and sleep disturbances should be given serious consideration. Psychosocial treatments have been shown to be effective for the treatment of all three of these conditions, and electroconvulsive therapy remains an effective treatment for major depression [21]. Exercise, simple behavioural strategies and environmental interventions have also been shown to be useful for enhancing sleep duration and quality.

Psychosocial therapies

The obvious adjunct to the pharmacological treatment and management of what are primarily psychological disorders is psychosocial therapy. There is now a great deal of evidence that a range of psychosocial therapies conducted by appropriately trained psychologists are very effective in treating anxiety, depression and insomnia in the general population [22–25], and increasing evidence that such approaches are also efficacious in older people [21,23,25] and clinical groups such as patients with coronary artery disease [26].

A large number of randomized clinical trials have established the efficacy of selected psychosocial interventions including cognitive behavioural therapy, and brief psychodynamic treatment for depression in older people [21, 31]. From their extensive review of this topic, Niederehe and Schneider concluded that in clinical practice, psychosocial treatments should be used in combination with pharmacological treatments and this ought to be considered standard care [21].

There are fewer studies on the effectiveness of treatments for later life anxiety disorders, and recommendations are based on findings from studies undertaken on younger persons, and older nonsymptomatic volunteers. The psychosocial treatments for anxiety that hold promise include relaxation methods, rational–emotive training and anxiety management training [21].

To maximize treatment efficacy, Niedre and Schneider recommend that comprehensive treatment 'packages' for anxiety and depression should be developed which integrate both psychological and biological components. These packages, however, should go beyond simply having the patient see the physician for medications and someone else for psychotherapy, but involve interdisciplinary collaboration in the primary care setting, and the inclusion of family members as key players in the overall treatment strategy [21].

Many behavioural interventions for insomnia have been undertaken and several reviews and meta-analyses of their effectiveness have been conducted [23–25]. Nowell et al. reviewed over 30 trials and concluded that stimulus control, i.e. instructional procedures designed to curtail incompatible sleep behaviours and regulate sleep–wake schedules, is an effective strategy for improving sleep quality [23]. These procedures are provided in Figure 14.2. Other effective strategies identified from the review include sleep restriction, relaxation, and cognitive behaviour therapy [23]. Similarly, Murtagh and Greenwood [24] and Morin et al. [25] found from their meta-analyses that psychological interventions produce reliable and durable benefits in the treatment of insomnia as determined by reduced sleep onset latency, increased sleep time, fewer nocturnal awakenings and improved sleep quality ratings. Morin et al. [25] also suggest that although psychological treatments may be more expensive and time-consuming than pharmacotherapy, they may be more cost-effective in the long term.

Simple behavioural strategies

In addition to structured psychosocial therapies, simple behavioural strategies such as avoiding stimulants (i.e. caffeine) in the evening and consuming a warm milk drink before bedtime may also assist sleep onset and quality. Taking a bath before bedtime has also been suggested as a mechanism for enhancing quality of sleep, particularly in older people. Kanda et al. [27] found that after bathing, the elderly people in their study were more likely to report good sleep and quicker sleep onset, verified by less frequent body movements in the first 3 hours of sleep. Older people may also benefit by simply being informed that they require less sleep than when they were younger, and that early waking in not unusual in older people [28].

Exercise

Another alternative to pharmacological therapy for sleep disturbances is the prescription of exercise, which has been found to have beneficial effects on sleep patterns in numerous recent studies [29–32]. Two randomized controlled trials have produced promising results in nursing home and community-dwelling older people. King et al. [30] evaluated the effect of a weekly, 30-minute moderate intensity exercise programme involving light aerobics and brisk walking in 67 sedentary

1. Go to bed only when sleepy.

2. Use the bed and bedroom only for sleep and sex (i.e. no reading, television watching, eating, or working during the day and night).

3. Get out of bed and go into another room whenever you are unable to sleep for 15-20 minutes and return only when sleepy again.

4. Arise in the morning at the same time regardless of the amount of sleep during the previous night.

5. Do not nap during the day.

Fig. 14.2.   Stimulus control therapy instructions for curtailing incompatible sleep behaviours and regulating sleep–wake schedules. From: Bootzin RR, Perlis ML. Non-pharmacological treatments of insomnia. *Journal of Clinical Psychiatry* 1992;53 (Suppl):37–41.

older community-dwelling subjects with moderate sleep complaints. Compared with the control group, the exercise group exhibited significant improvements in sleep quality and duration after the 16 weeks of exercise.

Physical activity also has a role to play in enhancing sleep among residents of aged care facilities. An investigation by Alessi et al. [32] assessed sleep quality and agitation in incontinent nursing home residents who were randomized to receive either (i) daytime physical activity and a night-time programme aimed at noise reduction (the intervention group), or (ii) night-time noise reduction programme only (the control group). Subjects who received the daytime activity experienced significantly improved sleep duration compared with those who received the night-time programme alone. Furthermore, 7 of the 15 intervention subjects had a decrease in observed agitation, compared with only 1 of the 14 control subjects.

Environmental interventions

Reducing light and noise and providing comfortable ambient temperatures are further 'sleep hygiene' approaches for enhancing sleep [33,34]. This is particularly important in acute hospitals to minimize the introduction of hypnotic medications to patients. This lessens the risk of patients falling while in hospital and maintaining use of these medications after hospital discharge. Providing an environment conducive to good sleep is also important in aged care residential facilities where the prevalence of hypnotic drug use is high.

Conclusion

The use of medications poses a significant risk for falling in older people, and as such, withdrawal or minimization of medication usage is an important component of a falls prevention programme. The available research suggests that withdrawal of antihypertensive medications is not warranted, as these drugs pose only a small increased falls risk and their withdrawal may have serious adverse effects on the conditions they were prescribed for. NSAID withdrawal is also unlikely to be of significant benefit, as these drugs also pose only a small increased falls risk, and their withdrawal may increase pain in subjects with osteoarthritis.

Withdrawal of psychoactive medications would appear to have the greatest potential as a falls prevention strategy, particularly in nursing homes. However, the available evidence suggests that while withdrawal of these drugs may be beneficial, limited compliance poses a major barrier to widespread utilization of this approach.

Psychosocial treatments are effective in the treatment of anxiety, depression and sleep disturbances in older people, and as such provide alternatives or complementary approaches to the pharmacological management of these conditions. Simple behavioural and environmental interventions and the prescription of exercise also offer additional means of enhancing sleep quality in this group.

REFERENCES

1 Atkin PA, Finegan TP, Ogle SJ, Talmont DM, Shenfield GM. Prevalence of drug-related admissions to a hospital geriatric service. *Australian Journal on Ageing* 1994;13:17–21.

2 Tinetti ME, Speechley M, Ginter SF. Risk factors for falls among elderly persons living in the community. *New England Journal of Medicine* 1988;319:1701–7.

3 Atkin PA, Ogle SJ, Finnegan TP, Shefield GM. Influence of 'academic detailing' on prescribing for elderly patients. *Health Promotion Journal of Australia* 1996;6:14–20.

4 Soumerai SB, Avorn J. Principles of educational outreach ('academic detailing') to improve clinical decision making. *Journal of the American Medical Association* 1990;263:549–56.

5 Avorn J, Soumerai SB. Improved drug-therapy decisions through educational outreach: a randomized controlled trial of academically based 'detailing'. *New England Journal of Medicine* 1983;308:1457–63.

6 Atkin PA, Finnegan TP, Ogle SJ, Shenfield GM. Are medication record cards useful ? *Medical Journal of Australia* 1995;162:300–1.

7 Bond WS, Schwartz M. Withdrawal reactions after long-term treatment with flurazepam. *Clinical Pharmacy* 1984;3:16–18.

8 Campbell AJ. Drug treatment as a cause of falls in old age. A review of the offending agents. *Drugs and Aging* 1991;1:289–302.

9 Avorn J, Soumerai SB, Everitt DE. A randomized controlled trial of a programme to reduce the use of psychoactive drugs in nursing homes. *New England Journal of Medicine* 1992;327:168–73.

10 Cumming RG. Epidemiology of medication-related falls and fractures in the elderly. *Drugs and Aging* 1998;12:43–53.

11 Yip YB, Cumming RG. The association between medications and falls in Australian nursing-home residents. *Medical Journal of Australia* 1994;160:14–18.

12 Curb JD, Applegate WB, Vogt TM. Antihypertensive therapy and falls and fractures in the Systolic Hypertension in the Elderly Program. *Journal of the American Geriatrics Society* 1993;41:SA15.

13 Campbell AJ, Robertson MC, Gardner MM, Norton RN, Buchner DM. Psychotropic medication withdrawal and a home-based exercise programme to prevent falls: results of a randomized controlled trial. *Journal of the American Geriatrics Society* 1999;47:850–3.

14 Gurwitz JH, Soumerai SB, Avorn J. Improving medication prescribing and utilization in the nursing home. *Journal of the American Geriatrics Society* 1990;38:542–52.

15 Ray WA, Meador KG, Taylor JA. Improving nursing home quality of care through provider education. *Annual Review of Gerontology and Geriatrics* 1992;12:183–204.

16 Rubenstein LZ, Robbins AS, Josephson KR, Schulman BL, Osterweil D. The value of assessing falls in an elderly population. A randomized clinical trial. *Annals of Internal Medicine* 1990;113:308–16.

17 Ray WA, Taylor JA, Meador KG, et al. A randomized trial of a consultation service to reduce falls in nursing homes. *Journal of the American Medical Association* 1997;278:557–62.

18 Bendall MJ, Bassey EJ, Pearson MB. Factors affecting walking speed of elderly people. *Age and Ageing* 1989;18:327–32.

19 Gibbs J, Hughes S, Dunlop D, Singer R, Chang RW. Predictors of change in walking velocity in older adults. *Journal of the American Geriatrics Society* 1996;44:126–32.

20 Stegman MR. Falls among elderly hypertensives: are they iatrogenic? *Gerontology* 1983;29:399–406.

21 Niederehe G, Schneider LS. Treatments for depression and anxiety in the aged. In: Nathan PE, Gorman JM: *A guide to treatments that work*. New York: Oxford University Press, 1998.

22 Brown C, Schulberg HC. The efficacy of psychosocial treatments in primary care: a review of randomized clinical trials. *General Hospital Psychiatry* 1995;17;414–24.

23 Nowell PD, Buysse DJ, Morin CM, Reynolds CF, Kupfer DJ. Effective treatments for selective sleep disorders. In Nathan PE, Gorman JM: *A guide to treatments that work*. New York: Oxford University Press, 1998.

24 Murtagh DR, Greenwood KM. Identifying effective psychological treatments for insomnia: a meta-analysis. *Journal of Consulting & Clinical Psychology* 1995;63:79–89.

25 Morin CM, Culbert JP, Schwartz SM. Nonpharmacological interventions for insomnia: a meta-analysis of treatment efficacy. *American Journal of Psychiatry* 1994;151:1172–80.

26 Linden W, Stossel C, Maurice J. Psychosocial interventions for patients with coronary artery disease: a meta-analysis. *Archives of Internal Medicine* 1996;156:745–52.

27 Kanda K, Tochihara Y, Ohnaka T. Bathing before sleep in the young and in the elderly. *European Journal of Applied Physiology and Occupational Physiology* 1999;80:71–5.

28 Morgan K. Sleep, insomnia and mental health. *Reviews in Clinical Gerontology* 1992;2:246–53.

29 Vitiello MV, Prinz PN, Schwartz RS. The subjective sleep quality of healthy older men and women is enhanced by participation in two fitness training programmes: a non-specific effect. *Sleep Research* 1994;23:148.

30 King AC, Oman RF, Brassington GS, Bliwise DL, Haskell WL. Moderate-intensity exercise and self-rated quality of sleep in older adults. A randomized controlled trial. *Journal of the American Medical Association* 1997;277:32–7.

31 Alessi CA, Schnelle JF, MacRae PG, et al. Does physical activity improve sleep in impaired nursing home residents? *Journal of the American Geriatrics Society* 1995;43:1098–102.

32 Alessi CA, Yoon EJ, Scnelle JF, Al-Samarrai NR, Cruise PA. A randomized controlled trial of a combined physical activity and environmental intervention in nursing home residents: do sleep and agitation improve? *Journal of the American Geriatrics Society* 1999;47:784–91.

33 Borkovec TD, Fowles DC. Controlled investigation of the effects of progressive and hypnotic relaxation of insomnia. *Journal of Abnormal Psychology* 1973;82:153–8.

34 Hauri P. Treating psychophysiological insomnia with biofeedback. *Archives of General Psychiatry* 1986;38:752–8.

15

Targeted falls prevention strategies

The previous chapters have focused primarily on strategies to address specific risk factors for falling. However, many older individuals have multiple falls risk factors. Within this population, people are also likely to have different combinations of risk factors. Therefore, a uniform intervention focusing on a specific factor may be too limited to address the multifactorial causes of falls in older people. Indeed, a number of authors have now designed and evaluated intervention programmes which involve assessment of risk and subsequent targeting of fall prevention strategies. These interventions are often made up of several of the strategies outlined in the Overview of Part II. This chapter seeks to outline and evaluate these studies.

Evaluation of targeted falls prevention strategies

A number of studies have now sought to evaluate targeted multifactorial intervention programmes. While it is common to look at the statistical significance of a difference between two or more groups in a study, additional useful information is obtained when the sizes of the effects of interventions are compared. The effect sizes of the key studies in this area are presented in Table 15.1, using a number of different methods. The proportions of fallers in each group (experimental and control group event rates), absolute risk reductions (the absolute difference between the control and experimental event rates), relative risk reduction (the difference between the event rates divided by the control group event rate), and the numbers needed to treat have been calculated for each of these studies. This approach is described by Sackett et al. [1]. The number needed to treat (NNT) describes the number of people who would need to undergo the intervention to prevent one fall and is the inverse of the relative risk reduction [1–3]. The studies in Table 15.1 are ranked by NNT. As the table shows, the numbers needed to treat for these interventions range from 5 to 25.

The methodological quality of studies should also be considered when conducting an evaluation of the effects of different interventions. In Table 15.1, these studies are rated for methodological quality using a rating scale developed as part

Table 15.1. Comparison of outcomes and quality of studies of targeted falls prevention programmes

Study	Follow-up period (months)	Control event rate (CER)	Experimental event rate (EER)	Relative risk reduction (RRR[a])	Absolute risk reduction (ARR[b])	Numbers needed to treat (NNT[c])	PEDro rating scale score (/11)
Close et al. 1999 [7]	12	52%	32%	38%	20%	5 people	6
Tinetti et al. 1994 [6]	12	47%	35%	26%	12%	8 people	8
Carpenter and Demopoulos 1990 [11]	36 [d, e]	19%	7%	63%	12%	8 people	5
Wagner et al. 1994 [8]	12	37%	28%	24%	9%	11 people	6
Fabacher et al. 1994 [12]	12	23%	14%	39%	9%	11 people	6
Hornbrook et al. 1994 [9]	23	44%	39%	11%	5%	20 people	6
Rubenstein et al. 1990 [16]	12	75%	71%	5%	4%	25 people	6

Notes:
[a] RRR = CER − EER/CER; [b] ARR = CER − EER; [c] NNT = 1/ARR; [d] falls data for 1-month period prior to survey; [e] data for total number of falls rather than number of fallers.

of the Physiotherapy Evidence Database (PEDro) project [4], which is based on a scale developed by Verhagen et al. [5]. As the table shows, there was little difference in the quality of the generally well-designed studies in this area. It should be noted that, while the maximum score on the scale is 11, this includes a total of three points for masking to group allocation. As these points are for masking of participants (not possible in these studies), those administering the intervention (not possible in these studies), and those assessing outcomes (not possible when self-reported falls risk is the key outcome), many studies in this area could only score a maximum of eight points.

A successful intervention programme was designed by Tinetti et al. [6]. This programme was trialled at the Yale site of the multicentre FICSIT trials (frailty and injuries: cooperative studies of intervention techniques). Interventions targeting risk factors identified at baseline assessment were compared with social visits.

Interventions included: medication adjustment, behavioural change recommendations, education and training, and home exercise programmes. During the 1-year follow-up phase, 47% of the control group fell compared with only 35% of the intervention group ($p = 0.04$). The adjusted incidence ratio for falling in the intervention group as compared with the control group was 0.69 (CI 0.52–0.90). Eight people would need to undergo this intervention for one fall to be prevented. This study was also of high methodological quality when rated on the PEDro scale.

A recent study by Close et al. [7] had an even greater effect size. Five people would need to undergo this intervention to prevent one fall. These authors found that a medical and occupational therapy assessment and subsequent tailored intervention resulted in a significant decrease in fall rates over a 1-year period. Participants in this study were people who had been seen at an Emergency Department following a fall. A substantial reduction in the risk of falling (OR 0.39, CI 0.23–0.66) and the risk of recurrent falls (OR 0.33, CI 0.16–0.68) was reported.

Another large randomized trial of a multifactorial falls prevention programme undertaken by Wagner et al. [8] showed some benefits of targeted intervention strategies. This study involved 1559 members of a health maintenance organization. One group received a nurse assessment home visit and follow-up interventions (targeting inadequate exercise, past falls, alcohol use, medication use, hearing and visual impairments). A second group received a general health promotion nurse visit and the third group received usual care. The intervention group experienced significantly fewer falls than the usual care group over the first year of follow-up. However, differences between the nurse assessment with follow-up intervention group and the general health promotion nurse visit group were not significant. Benefits were not well maintained in the second year of follow-up with no difference in falling rates between the groups at this time. This suggests the need for ongoing monitoring of and intervention for falls risk factors.

Several falls prevention programmes have used group education sessions. In a randomized trial involving 3182 independently living health maintenance organization members aged 65 and over, Hornbrook et al. [9], found that a home assessment and advice on modifications followed by a group education, exercise and discussion programme, reduced falls by 11%. This intervention was somewhat less effective than the more targeted interventions described above, with 20 people needing to receive the intervention to prevent one fall. Furthermore, Reinsch et al. [10] found that a general nontargeted education programme involving classes on exercise, relaxation and health and safety topics was not effective in preventing falls among community-dwellers attending senior citizens centres.

There is also some evidence of the efficacy of home-based health and disability screening for older people. While these programmes have broader aims than reducing falls they can involve the identification of risk factors for falling. Carpenter and

Demopoulos [11] conducted a randomized trial involving 539 people aged 75 and over. The intervention group were visited and assessed by volunteers at regular intervals. Participants who developed increasing disability were referred to their family doctor for interventions as required. The number of falls reported by the control group doubled between the first and last interview but remained the same for the intervention group. However, another study [12] found only a trend to a decreased falls rate following one screening visit by a physician's assistant or nurse then two follow-up visits by trained volunteers. Potential problems identified by the screening tool were addressed with referral and/or advice. The screening visit was followed by a letter outlining findings and recommendations. Despite the lack of statistical significance, this study found a 39% decrease in falls among the intervention group and calculations show that 11 people would need to undergo the intervention to prevent one fall.

Falls assessment clinics which aim to identify and modify falls risk factors among those who have already fallen have been suggested as a falls prevention strategy [13–15]. To evaluate this approach among residents of a long-term residential care facility, Rubenstein et al. [16] conducted a randomized clinical trial of a specialized post-fall medical assessment (compared with usual care) among 160 ambulatory older people. The assessment involved identification and recommendation for treatment of various falls risk factors (e.g. weakness, environmental hazards, orthostatic hypotension, drug side effects, gait problems). The 9% reduction in falls among the intervention group over 2 years was not statistically significant. However, the intervention group did experience significantly fewer hospital admissions and shorter hospital stays.

Several of these studies which did not show a difference in falls rates may have lacked the statistical power to detect a difference. This may be overcome by combining the results of individual studies in a meta-analysis. Indeed, when the results of five studies of targeted falls and fracture prevention strategies [6, 8, 12, 16, 17] were pooled as part of the Cochrane Collaboration review [18], the results suggested 'that an intervention in which older people are assessed by a health professional trained to identify intrinsic and environmental risk factors is likely to reduce the number of people sustaining falls (OR 0.79; 95% CI 0.65–0.96)'. The authors also report that 'although not quite reaching statistical significance, the number sustaining a fall requiring medical care (OR 0.70; 95% CI 0.47–1.04), and the number sustaining a fall resulting in injury (OR 0.73; 95% CI 0.51–1.04) may also be reduced'.

Conclusion

Now that a number of large prospective studies have conclusively determined key risk factors for falling, it seems that the multifaceted programmes should involve targeting of interventions to an individual's problems rather than offering the same intervention to all. Indeed, a number of well-designed studies have shown the potential benefits of a range of targeted multifaceted falls prevention programmes, with between 5 and 25 people needing to be treated to prevent one fall. While not all studies have shown targeted multifaceted falls prevention programmes are effective, pooling of data shows a significant effect on reducing falls. However, as this has involved the pooling of studies which involve quite different interventions, further investigation of the effects of particular approaches to targeting intervention is required.

Unfortunately, a mutifaceted approach makes it difficult to assess the relative effects of different programmes and their components. Furthermore, factorial designs and individual programmes also need continued investigation to establish which components of the multifaceted package are necessary. This area of falls prevention research is changing rapidly. There have been several trials of this type published in recent years, and many more are currently under way. When these findings become available, a clearer picture of effective intervention components and optimal mutifactorial approaches will emerge.

REFERENCES

1 Sackett D, Richardson W, Rosenberg W, Haynes R. *Evidence-based medicine: how to practice and teach EBM.* Edinburgh: Churchill Livingstone, 1998.

2 Chatellier G, Zapletal E, LeMaitre D, Menard J, Degoulet P. The Number Needed to Treat: a clinically useful nomogram in its proper context. *British Medical Journal* 1996;312:426–9.

3 Laupacis A, Sackett D, Roberts R. An assessment of clinically useful measures of the consequences of treatment. *New England Journal of Medicine* 1988;318:1728–33.

4 Herbert R, Moseley A, Sherrington C. PEDro: a database of randomized controlled trials in physiotherapy. *Health Information Management* 1999;28:186–8.

5 Verhagen A, de Vet H, de Bie R, et al. The Delphi list: a criteria list for quality assessment of randomized clinical trials for conducting systematic reviews developed by Delphi consensus. *Journal of Clinical Epidemiology* 1998;51:1235–41.

6 Tinetti ME, Baker DI, McAvay G, et al. A multifactorial intervention to reduce the risk of falling among elderly people living in the community. *New England Journal of Medicine* 1994;331:821–7.

7 Close J, Ellis M, Hooper R, Glucksman E, Jackson S, Swift C. Prevention of falls in the elderly trial (PROFET): a randomized controlled trial. *Lancet* 1999;353:93–7.

8 Wagner EH, LaCroix AZ, Grothaus L, et al. Preventing disability and falls in older adults: a population-based randomized trial. *American Journal of Public Health* 1994;84:1800–6.

9 Hornbrook MC, Stevens VJ, Wingfield DJ, Hollis JF, Greenlick MR, Ory MG. Preventing falls among community-dwelling older persons: results from a randomized trial. *Gerontologist* 1994;34:16–23.

10 Reinsch S, MacRae P, Lachenbruch PA, Tobis JS. Attempts to prevent falls and injury: a prospective community study. *Gerontologist* 1992;32:450–6.

11 Carpenter G, Demopoulos G. Screening the elderly in the community: controlled trial of dependency surveillance using a questionnaire administered by volunteers. *British Medical Journal* 1990;300:1253–6.

12 Fabacher D, Josephson K, Pietruszka F, Linderborn K, Morley J, Rubenstein L. An in-home preventive assessment programme for independent older adults. *Journal of the American Geriatrics Society* 1994;42:630–8.

13 Wolf-Klein GP, Silverstone FA, Basavaraju N, Foley CJ, Pascaru A, Ma PH. Prevention of falls in the elderly population. *Archives of Physical Medicine and Rehabilitation* 1988;69:689–91.

14 Hill KD, Dwyer JM, Schwarz JA, Helme RD. A falls and balance clinic for the elderly. *Physiotherapy Canada* 1994;46:20–7.

15 Tideiksaar R. Reducing the risk of falls and injury in older persons: contribution of a falls and immobility clinic. In: Lafont C, Baroni A, Allard M, et al., editors. *Facts and research in gerontology. Falls, gait and balance disorders in the elderly: from successful aging to frailty.* New York: Springer, 1996:163–82.

16 Rubenstein LZ, Robbins AS, Josephson KR, Schulman BL, Osterweil D. The value of assessing falls in an elderly population. A randomized clinical trial. *Annals of Internal Medicine* 1990;113:308–16.

17 Vetter NJ, Lewis PA, Ford D. Can health visitors prevent fractures in elderly people? *British Medical Journal* 1992;304:888–90.

18 Gillespie LD, Gillespie WJ, Cumming R, Lamb SE, Rowe BH. Interventions for preventing falls in the elderly (Cochrane Review). The Cochrane Library, issue 3. Oxford: Update Software, 1999.

16

A physiological profile approach for falls prevention

As indicated in Chapter 15, a major conclusion from the Cochrane Collaboration's systematic review on falls prevention was that protection against falling may be maximized by interventions which target multiple, identified risk factors in individual patients and that health care providers should consider health screening of at-risk elderly people, followed by targeted interventions for deficit areas [1]. Consistent with this conclusion, we have developed a falls risk assessment which makes use of normative data from large population studies to identify older people with impairments in one or more of the major physiological domains that have been shown to be risk factors for falls – information which makes it possible to make specific recommendations for preventing falls on an individual basis. This chapter outlines the nature and elements of this assessment and describes a randomized controlled trial that is using this assessment to identify appropriate interventions for older people at risk of falls.

The physiological profile assessment for assessing falls risk

The physiological profile assessment (PPA) has two versions: a comprehensive or long version and a screening or short version. The comprehensive version is suitable for rehabilitation, physical therapy and occupational therapy settings and for dedicated falls clinics, and takes 45 minutes to administer. The screening version takes 10–15 minutes to administer and is suitable for acute hospitals and long-term care institutions. Table 16.1 describes the PPA test items for the comprehensive version. The screening version contains five of these items: a test of vision (edge contrast sensitivity), peripheral sensation (proprioception), lower limb strength (knee extension strength), reaction time using a finger press as the response and body sway (sway when standing on medium density foam rubber). These five items were identified from discriminant analyses as being the most important for discriminating between fallers and nonfallers [2, 3]. The physiological profile assessment tests are described in Table 16.1 and illustrated in Figures 16.1–16.7.

For inclusion in the PPA, the tests had to meet a number of criteria. First, tests

Table 16.1. The physiological profile assessment tests

Test	Test description
High-and low-contrast visual acuity	Visual acuity is measured using a chart with high-contrast visual acuity letters (similar to a Snellen scale) and low-contrast (10%) letters, (where contrast = the difference between the maximum and minimum luminances divided by their sum). Acuity is assessed binocularly with subjects wearing their spectacles (if needed) at a test distance of 3m and measured in terms of the minimum angle resolvable (MAR) in minutes of arc.
Contrast sensitivity	Edge contrast sensitivity is assessed using the Melbourne Edge Test. This test presents 20 circular patches containing edges with reducing contrast. Correct identification of the orientation of the edges on the patches provides a measure of contrast sensitivity in decibel units, where $dB = -10\log_{10}$ contrast.
Visual field dependence	The visual field dependence test places vision and vestibular and other postural cues in conflict. Subjects attempt to align a straight edge to the true vertical while exposed to a rotating visual stimulus which extends over most of the visual field. Errors in aligning the rod to the true vertical are measured in degrees.
Tactile sensitivity	Tactile sensitivity is measured with a pressure aesthesiometer. This instrument contains eight nylon filaments of equal length, but varying in diameter. The filaments are applied to the centre of the lateral malleolus and measurements are expressed in logarithms of milligrams pressure.
Vibration sense	Vibration sense is measured using an electronic device which generates a 200 Hz vibration of varying intensity. The vibration is applied to the tibial tuberosity and is measured in microns of motion perpendicular to the body surface.
Proprioception	Proprioception is assessed by asking seated subjects with eyes closed to align the lower limbs on either side of a 60×60 cm by 1-cm-thick clear acrylic sheet standing on edge and inscribed with a protractor. Any difference in matching the great toes is measured in degrees.
Lower limb strength	The strength of three leg muscle groups (knee flexors and extensors and ankle dorsiflexors) is measured while subjects are seated. In each test, there are three trials and the greatest force is recorded.
Reaction time	Reaction time is assessed using a light as the stimulus and depression of a switch (by either the finger or the foot) as the response. Reaction time is measured in milliseconds.

Table 16.1. (*cont.*)

Test	Test description
Postural sway	Sway is measured using a sway meter that measures displacements of the body at waist level. The device consists of a 40-cm-long rod with a vertically mounted pen at its end. The rod is attached to subjects by a firm belt and extends posteriorly. As subjects attempt to stand as still as possible, the pen records the sway of subjects on a sheet of millimetre graph paper fastened to the top of an adjustable height table. Testing is performed with the eyes open and closed while standing on a firm surface and on a piece of medium-density foam rubber (15 cm thick). Total sway (number of millimetre squares traversed by the pen) in the 30-second periods is recorded for the four tests.

were required to assess all of the major physiological systems that contribute to balance control. In addition the tests needed to be simple to administer, of short duration, and feasible for older people to undertake. They also needed to provide valid and reliable measurements, be 'low tech', robust and portable, and be capable of providing quantitative measurements. The rationale for these criteria is outlined below.

1 *Simple to administer:* To enable widespread use of the assessment, each test needs to be simple to administer. Thus, only minimal training is required before personnel become proficient in test administration.

2 *Short administration time:* To test the many domains important in balance control in one session, it is important that each individual test item does not take too long to administer. Quick administration time aids participation, and avoids fatigue in frail older people.

3 *Feasible for older people to undertake:* The selected tests need to be acceptable to older people, in that they need to be noninvasive and not require excessive effort or cause pain or discomfort. None the less, the tests need to be challenging so as to discriminate between older people with and without sensorimotor and balance impairments.

4 *Valid and reliable measurements:* The tests must have high criterion validity, that is, they can predict falling in older people. When combined in multivariate discriminant analyses, these tests can predict those at risk of falling with 75% accuracy in both community and institutional settings [2–4]. They also have high test–retest and interrater reliability [5].

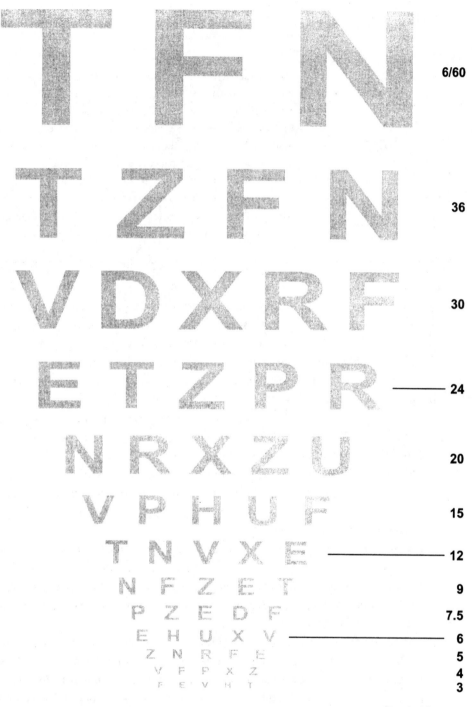

Read at 3m

Fig. 16.1.   The low contrast visual acuity test.

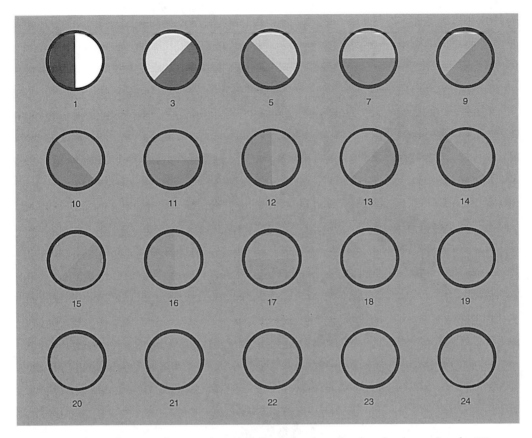

Fig. 16.2.   The Melbourne Edge Test. (Permission to reproduce the chart has been given by J.H. Verbaken.)

5 *'Low tech' and robust:* If the tests are to be used successfully in community settings, they need to be 'low tech' and robust.

6 *Portability:* Compact, lightweight test apparatus enables portability of the assessment clinic. Thus, assessment clinics can be set up on a temporary or permanent basis in community settings, retirement villages, and healthcare institutions. This improves participation and compliance, as the laboratory can be brought to the target population of often frail older people, rather than relying on them attending a fixed position laboratory.

7 *Quantitative measurements:* Finally, a fundamental criterion for each test is that it provides continuously scored measurements rather than discrete or graded scores. This enables the test measures to be analysed by powerful parametric statistics, such as analysis of variance, correlation and regression techniques and discriminant analysis. The tests are standardized and minimize subjective judgement on the part of the test administrator. The quantitative measures also avoid

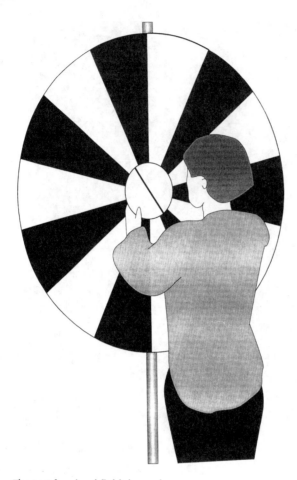

Fig. 16.3.   The test for visual field dependence.

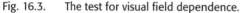

ceiling and floor effects, which can be quite common in subjective assessments
of vision, sensation, strength and balance.

For both the short and long forms, a computer program has been developed to
assess an individual's performance in relation to a normative database compiled
from large population studies [3, 4]. (This program can be viewed on the Internet
at www.powmri.unsw.edu.au/FBRG/FBRGhome.htm. Along with the test items
required for performing the PPA, the program can be obtained by contacting the
authors.) The programme produces a falls risk assessment report for each individual and includes the following four components:

1 A graph indicating an individual's overall falls risk score.
2 A profile of the individual's test performances. This allows a quick identification
   of physiological strengths and weaknesses.

(a)

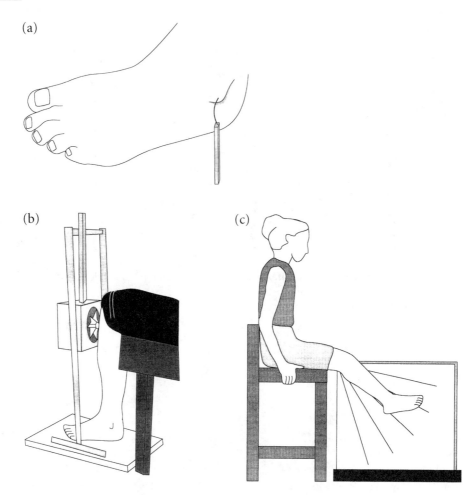

(b)   (c)

Fig. 16.4.   Peripheral sensation tests: (a) tactile sensitivity, (b) vibration sense, (c) proprioception.

3 A table indicating the individual's test performances in relation to age-matched norms.

4 A written report which explains the results and makes recommendations for improving functional performances and compensating for any impairments identified.

A falls risk graph for a 70-year-old women is shown in Figure 16.8. The falls risk score is a single index score derived from a discriminant function analysis that was found to discriminate accurately between elderly fallers and nonfallers in large population studies [2–4]. This graph presents the falls risk score in relation to persons of the same age and in relation to falls risk criteria ranging from very low to marked.

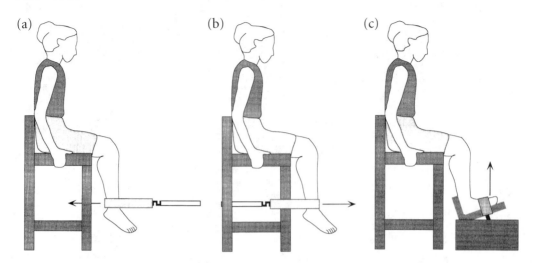

Fig. 16.5.   Strength tests: (a) knee flexors, (b) knee extensors, (c) ankle dorsiflexors.

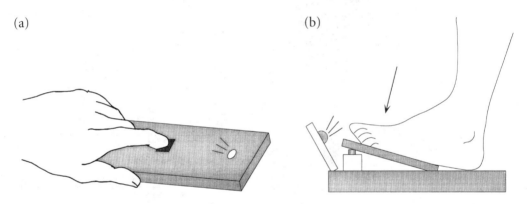

Fig. 16.6.   Reaction time tests: (a) finger press, (b) foot press.

The profile of test performance results presents an individual's scores in each test in relation to population norms in standard (z score) format. Thus, a score of zero indicates an average performance, positive scores indicate above average performances and negative scores indicate below average performances. Each unit represents one standard deviation. As the scores have been standardized, the test results can be compared with each other. Figure 16.9 shows an example of the comprehensive version PPA profile.

The table of individual test performances in relation to young normal and age- and sex-matched norms from the comprehensive version of the PPA is shown in Figure 16.10. This presents the results of the tests in a conventional manner and complements the test performance profile graph.

Finally, the computer programme compiles a written report for each individual.

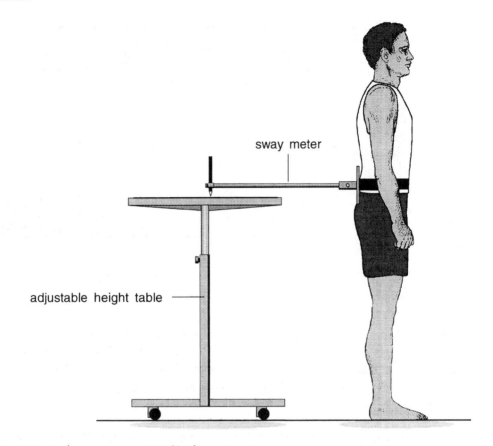

sway meter

adjustable height table

Fig. 16.7.   Postural sway assessment using the sway meter.

An example is presented in Figure 16.11; it summarizes the findings, highlights below-average performances and makes individual recommendations for reducing falls risk.

Using the PPA to optimize falls prevention strategies in at-risk older people: a randomized controlled trial

At present, we are conducting a randomized controlled falls prevention trial involving 600 community-dwelling persons aged 75 years and over. The major aim is to determine whether tailored interventions (identified by the comprehensive PPA) can reduce the rate of falling in older community-dwelling people by maximizing functional performance in the following physiological domains: strength, balance, vision, peripheral sensation, vestibular function and visual field dependence.

Subjects allocated to the intervention group in this study receive their

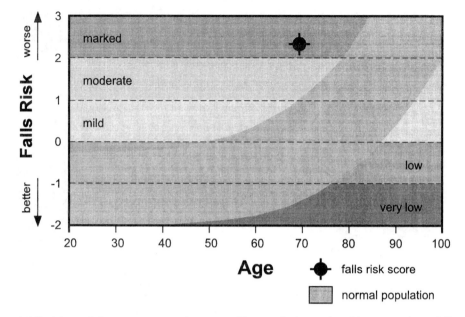

Fig. 16.8.   A falls risk graph for a woman aged 70 years. The graph shows that this woman has a falls risk score of 2.37, which indicates she has a marked risk of falling. Her score is also above the curved band which depicts the age-related falls-risk normal band. This indicates her score is higher than would be expected for women of her age.

computer-generated falls risk report. Its four components are explained and depending on the test results, the following interventions are arranged.

1 Exercise interventions for improving strength, coordination and balance.
2 Appropriate surgical, optical and behavioural interventions for maximizing vision.
3 A counselling intervention on strategies to compensate for reduced peripheral sensation.
4 A counselling intervention on strategies to compensate for reduced vestibular function and increased visual field dependence.

Brief descriptions of the interventions are provided below.

The exercise intervention

Subjects who perform poorly in the tests of strength, reaction time and balance are allocated to this intervention. They then take part in 1-hour exercise classes twice a week for 12 months. Instructors experienced in conducting exercise programmes for older people lead these exercise classes. In addition to some core balance, strength and coordination exercises, subjects complete individual exercise regimes based on their falls risk profiles: subjects with muscle weakness in specific muscle

Test	Z-score	-3	-2	-1	0	1	2	3
Visual acuity (high contrast)	-1.48							
Visual acuity (low contrast)	-2.01							
Edge contrast sensitivity	-1.73							
Visual field dependence	0.74							
Proprioception	0.51							
Tactile sensitivity - ankle	0.89							
Vibration sense - knee	0.3							
Ankle dorsiflexion strength	-0.25							
Knee extension strength	0.12							
Knee flexion strength	-0.51							
Reaction time hand	-0.14							
Reaction time foot	0.05							
Sway on floor - eyes open	-1.02							
Sway on floor - eyes closed	-0.88							
Sway on foam - eyes open	-1.87							
Sway on foam - eyes closed	-2.05							

Fig. 16.9.   The test performance profile for the woman whose falls risk graph is shown in Figure 16.8. The bars show performance in each test in relation to norms for persons aged 60 years and over. Scores above zero indicate above average performances and scores below zero indicate below average performances (as derived from population norms for persons aged 65 years and over). Scores <-1 indicate functionally important impairments. The profile shows good performances in the tests of peripheral sensation and visual field dependence, average performances in the tests of strength and reaction time, and below average performances in the tests of vision and balance. For this individual, interventions would be aimed at improving vision and balance.

groups receive specific exercises to improve their strength; those with poor balance receive task-specific balance training; and those who performed poorly in the simple and choice reaction time tests take part in exercises that challenge speed and coordination. The exercises are held in classes so as to monitor accurately attendance and compliance.

The visual intervention

Subjects with poor vision allocated to visual intervention are referred to an ophthalmologist to assess the need for new spectacles and/or cataract surgery. The subjects also receive counselling which includes advices on wearing spectacles, avoiding dimly lit areas, taking special care when walking outside at night or at dusk, and making sure to turn the light on at night for visits to the toilet, etc. On the basis of

TEST RESULTS

Measure	Score	Young normal	Age-matched~
Vision			
Visual acuity (high contrast)	2.5**	(0.54 - 0.82)	(0.83 - 1.58)
Visual acuity (low contrast)	6**	(0.76 - 1.05)	(1.32 - 2.65)
Edge contrast sensitivity	13**	(23 - 24)	(20 - 24)
Visual field dependence	1.5	(0.0 - 2.0)	(0.5 - 6.5)
Sensation			
Proprioception	1	(0.2 - 1.4)	(0.4 - 2.4)
Tactile sensitivity - ankle	3.7	(3.22 - 4.08)	(3.61 - 4.31)
Vibration sense - knee	15.5	(2 - 5)	(7 - 34)
Strength			
Ankle dorsiflexion strength	7	(10 - 15)	(6 - 10.5)
Knee extension strength	21	(35 - 58)	(15 - 29)
Knee flexion strength	10	(22 - 29)	(10 - 17)
Speed and Control			
Reaction time - hand	251	(182 - 236)	(197 - 267)
Reaction time - foot	278	(213 - 273)	(230 - 305)
Balance			
Sway on floor - eyes open	120**	(35 - 70)	(40 - 100)
Sway on floor - eyes closed	158	(55 - 95)	(50 - 160)
Sway on foam - eyes open	286**	(60-110)	(65 - 163)
Sway on foam - eyes closed	581**	(70 - 185)	(108 - 285)

~ Women aged 70-74 years.
# Better than average age-matched (i.e. top 10%).
** Worse than average age-matched.

Fig. 16.10.   The table of individual test results for the woman whose falls risk graph is shown in Figure 16.8. The table presents the raw test results, and compares the individual's test performances to young normal performances and age- and sex-matched normative performances. Scores marked with dual asterisks indicate performances below that expected for a person of that age and sex.

the test results and ophthalmological referral, one or more of the following interventions are implemented, as required: (i) the provision of single-focus spectacles with the appropriate visual correction, (ii) the provision of two sets of spectacles; one pair with the appropriate visual correction and another pair for reading, so as to stop use of bifocal spectacles when moving around, and (iii) cataract surgery.~

The peripheral sensation counselling intervention

Subjects are informed about how lower limb sensation provides information about position and movement and the role reduced lower limb sensation plays in impairing balance. Subjects are advised to: (i) take particular care when walking on irregular or soft surfaces such as uneven ground and carpets; (ii) use a walking stick or a light cane as a sensor (rather than/or in addition to a support) to compensate for sensation loss; and (iii) wear shoes with low heels and firm rubber soles. Subjects

21 September 1999

Jane Smith
10 Union St
Sydney NSW 2000

Dear Mrs Smith,

Please find attached the report regarding your balance assessment at Prince of Wales Medical Research Institute on 21 September, 1999. These test results indicate that you have an increased risk of falling.

You performed well in the important test/s of visual field dependence, proprioception, and tactile sensitivity. In some areas however, you were below average for your age group, so the following recommendations may be of help to you.

One or more of your vision tests was below average. Reduced vision can increase the risk of a trip over an unseen object in the environment such as steps, gutters and footpath cracks and raised edges. It is recommended that you should see an eye specialist for an assessment if you have not done so in the past year. You may also benefit by wearing a single lens pair of glasses, especially when outside. It is recommended that you do not wear bifocal or multifocal spectacles, as the lower sections of these spectacles blur items at critical distances on the ground and this can lead to trips. Wearing a hat when outside also improves vision by reducing glare substantially.

Your sway scores were high indicating reduced balance control. There are certain situations where you should take particular care: when walking on soft or uneven surfaces such as thick carpets and soft or rough ground. You may also be at risk of losing balance in dim or unlit areas, so avoid such areas where possible and make sure you turn the light on before walking in the house at night. Exercises can improve strength, co-ordination and balance. It is recommended that you increase your current level of physical activity, with a program of planned walks three times a week and a complementary program of group or home-based exercises. The attached home exercises could benefit you in this area. Finally, it is recommended that you wear shoes with low heels and firm rubber soles. These are best for balance.
For enquiries regarding this report, please contact the Falls Risk Assessment Program at Prince of Wales Medical Research Institute on 9999-9999.

Yours sincerely,

Dr Anthony Jones

Fig. 16.11.   An example of the written report compiled by the PPA computer programme.

with marked sensation loss are also referred to their general practitioner to assess whether any medical condition such as diabetes could be leading to the sensory loss.

The vestibular system and visual field dependence counselling intervention

Information is given to subjects explaining that their score in the field dependence test (a test which places vision in conflict with proprioception and vestibular sense) indicates that they are particularly reliant on their vision for information about the upright. They are advised to attend to objects in the environment that are known to be vertical and stationary, such as door frames when inside the house and buildings when outside. It is stressed that this is especially important when they are near moving vehicles and in crowded, busy places (visually complex areas) such as shopping centres and busy roads.

To determine the effectiveness of the programme the intervention and control subjects will be reassessed for the physiological measures at six months, and all subjects will be followed up for falls for a 12-month period after the initial assessment. A full evaluation of the costs and cost-effectiveness of the programme will also be undertaken as part of the project. The study is planned for completion in 2001.

Conclusion

There is increasing evidence that multifaceted intervention programmes can reduce the risk of falling in older people. In particular, intervention programmes that identify specific risk factors and intervene accordingly may offer maximum protection against falls. The use of population norms to identify poor performances in the diverse array of physiological domains involved in balance control offers an insightful means for initiating appropriate and effective interventions. The findings of a large randomized controlled trial, currently under way, should determine whether this physiological profile-based approach is effective in preventing falls in older community-dwelling people.

REFERENCES

1 Gillespie LD, Gillespie WJ, Cumming R, Lamb SE, Rowe BH. Interventions for preventing falls in the elderly (Cochrane Review). The Cochrane Library, issue 3. Oxford: Update Software, 1999.

2 Lord SR, Clark RD, Webster IW. Physiological factors associated with falls in an elderly population. *Journal of the American Geriatrics Society* 1991;39:1194–200.

3 Lord SR, Ward JA, Williams P, Anstey KJ. Physiological factors associated with falls in older community-dwelling women. *Journal of the American Geriatrics Society* 1994;42:1110–17.

4 Lord SR, Sambrook PN, Gilbert C, et al. Postural stability, falls and fractures in the elderly: results from the Dubbo osteoporosis epidemiology study. *Medical Journal of Australia* 1994; 160:684–5,688–91.

5 Lord SR, Castell S. The effect of a physical activity programme on balance, strength, neuro-muscular control and reaction time in older persons. *Archives of Physical Medicine and Rehabilitation* 1994;75:648–52.

Part III

Research issues in falls prevention

17

Falls in older people: future directions for research

Since the pioneering work of Sheldon in the 1960s, a great deal of research has been undertaken into falls and there is now a considerable body of knowledge about the various risk factors and the effectiveness of a range of intervention strategies. However, as in every area of scientific study, it is often the case that the findings of one study pose questions for another. In this final chapter, we present a brief review of a range of research issues that need to be addressed in the future.

Studies on human balance and related sensorimotor systems

Further studies are required to enhance our understanding of human balance. In particular, further work is needed to elucidate whether impairments in vestibular functioning that lead to a reduced sense of the upright, and/or unstable retinal images during head movements are significant causes of falling in older people. Contributions from the vestibular system to dynamic balance and gait also need clarification. Similarly, more precise tests of vision are required to identify specific visual functions that are particularly important for avoiding falls. Further research is also required into complex factors such as responses to postural disturbances and the planning and execution of functional activities such as standing up, stepping, walking, stair-climbing and obstacle avoidance.

Transient risk factors

As indicated in Part I of this book, most headway into identifying risk factors for falls has been in the area of chronic conditions. New studies are required to tackle the more difficult areas of transient falls risk factors. The main areas that require attention in this regard are cardiovascular conditions including orthostatic hypotension and disorders of vestibular function. This may best be achieved by integrated approaches to the investigation of dizziness and syncope; however, before any real progress can be made in this area, a clearer consensus needs to be reached regarding the very definitions of these terms. As discussed in Chapter 5, progress towards a more complete understanding of dizziness is considerably hampered by inconsistent definitions across the literature [1].

Another area which has received only limited attention is the evaluation of the mechanisms underlying transient loss of balance in response to certain medications. While one recent study reported a dose-dependent increase in sway in response to psychoactive medication use [2], further work is required to assess how different medications impair stability when performing more complex tasks, and the duration of this impairment.

Neuropsychological risk factors

Authors have recently included neuropsychological assessments in their studies of balance control and their screening batteries for predicting falls [3,4]. Choice reaction time tasks, and other speeded tests have proved to be good discriminators between fallers and nonfallers [3,5,6]. Measures of impulsivity and ability to perform dual tasks have also been found to be associated with balance and falls [4,7]. While poor performance in these tests may indicate general cognitive decline, they provide interesting insights into the causes of falls. Intervention strategies aimed at increasing psychomotor speed and reducing impulsivity and 'risk-taking' behaviour in older people would be an exciting endeavour.

Falls prevention in population subgroups

Chapter 4 outlined the many medical conditions that predispose older people to falling. Studies identifying means of improving physical functioning are required in these population subgroups. Development of intervention programmes for the following patient groups would be important in this regard: persons with Parkinson's disease or dementia and those who have suffered a hip fracture or stroke.

Intensity and type of exercise intervention programmes

Further work is required to identify the most effective exercise interventions for improving physical functioning and preventing falls in older people. The grouped results from the FICSIT studies [8] indicated that intervention studies that addressed strength alone were ineffective in preventing falls, whereas studies that included a balance component achieved reductions in falling rates. This needs to be corroborated in further studies. There is no doubt that as the older population comprises a diverse group in relation to physical functioning, there will be no single exercise prescription for this group. Specific studies are required to identify exercise components that are effective in maintaining strength, coordination, and balance and the ability to carry out functional activities in both the more vigorous, independent older population and in frailer groups. Exercise studies also need to be conducted as public health interventions, not just as demonstration projects, to identify programmes that are acceptable to older people in the long term. Such work should also address strategies for overcoming barriers to exercise participation.

Optimal shoe designs

Chapter 10 synthesized the available information gleaned from studies undertaken to date. There is no doubt that high-heeled shoes constitute a needless falls risk factor for older women. Other posited hazardous and safe shoe characteristics still require evaluating in appropriate experimental and prospective epidemiological studies. In particular, the following areas require investigation: heel collar height, sole flare, tread patterns and sole hardness. Further, studies are required to determine whether there is one optimal shoe type for older persons for all circumstances or whether there are shoe characteristics that are particularly suited to certain conditions. For example, it needs to be determined whether a shoe that is appropriate for wearing indoors is also appropriate for wearing outdoors. Studies are also required to identify the shoe characteristics that maximize balance in situations that predispose people to falls, such as wet and slippery floors and uneven and soft ground.

Preventing falls in institutions

The major risk factors for falls for older persons in acute hospitals and nursing homes have been identified. Multidisciplinary, multifactorial assessment and intervention programmes addressing these risk factors now need to be fully evaluated for their efficacy and cost-effectiveness in research trials. The effectiveness of specific interventions such as patient movement alarms, alterations to bed heights and use or nonuse of cot sides also needs to be determined. Furthermore, staffing issues need to be fully assessed to determine whether modifications to timetabling of nursing and support staff can increase vigilance and identify potential hazards in the institutional environment.

Home modifications

As discussed in Chapter 9, the study by Cumming et al. [9] suggests that an occupational therapy intervention which involves home hazard assessment and modification, as well as advice on footwear and safety behaviour may be effective in preventing falls, particularly in those with a history of falls. Further research is required to determine whether home modification alone can prevent falls.

Interventions for modifying medication use

As indicated in Chapter 5, the role of many medications as risk factors for falls may have been overstated. In many cases, it appears that medication use has simply been a marker for the medical conditions for which they were prescribed. The psycho-active medications, however, have been consistently shown to be significant and independent risk factors for falls. In the recent well-planned and executed study, Campbell et al. [10] found that it is extremely difficult to recruit older users of psychoactive medications into a study aimed at terminating their use. Further, it proved difficult to modify psychoactive medication use in the minority who did participate. Further work is required to identify alternatives to pharmacological treatment of sleep disorders and anxiety in older people. As benzodiazepine with-drawal, in particular, has been shown to be difficult, strategies for preventing initial use of these medications would be important to identify. To be successful, such strategies would need to be seen as an acceptable alternative to medication use by older people and by their doctors and other health professionals.

Intervention compliance

Regardless of the intervention modality for preventing falls, a crucial factor is com-pliance. There is a growing body of knowledge of factors related to adherence to exercise. Further work is required to determine if similar factors also predict poor compliance to other interventions such as medication withdrawal, use of hip pro-tectors and adoption of home safety modifications.

Evaluation of falls clinics

The past 10 years has seen the advent of falls clinics [11, 12]. These have been devised on an individual basis with no two clinics alike. The main models, however, have included (i) clinics which use a standardized protocol for the medical man-agement of falls; (ii) clinics which involve the contributions of pertinent health professionals such as different medical specialists, physiotherapists, occupational therapists and podiatrists and (iii) clinics which use screening tests for identifying those at risk of falling and the underlying impairments, with intervention strate-gies targeted to identified deficit areas. These clinics still require evaluation with respect to their effectiveness and cost-effectiveness compared with usual care.

Multifactorial targeted interventions

Studies are required which accurately identify falls risk factors and target interventions to the identified deficit areas. To achieve this, appropriate screening assessments are required, and specific proven interventions put in place to maximize physical functioning and minimize falls risk on an individual basis. A simple screening procedure linked with effective public health interventions may offer great scope for reducing fall rates in at-risk older people.

Determining the best interventions

There are now some encouraging findings from well-planned and executed studies which indicate that many falls are preventable. Multifactorial interventions, in particular, have shown promise in this regard. However, further work is still required to determine which interventions are the most effective, and whether some interventions may actually cause harm. This evidence will only be provided by randomized controlled trials, particularly those with factorial designs, and their meta-analyses. However, as the causes of falls are multifactorial and the older population is a diverse one, there is likely to be no single formula for preventing falls. Further, in the case of particular intervention modalities such as exercise, it is likely that alternatives are required to provide effective and acceptable options for older people to adopt and adhere to. Certain 'common sense' interventions such as reducing hazards in the home, still require corroboration from carefully executed epidemiological studies.

Conclusion

Falls and falls-related injury are likely to be major healthcare problems for older people for the foreseeable future. Consequently, the identification and implementation of effective falls prevention strategies will remain an important public health priority. Much has been learned about risk factors for falls and fractures in recent years, but further work remains to be done to understand fully the role of certain medical, physiological and environmental factors in predisposing older people to falls. Currently, known effective interventions include physical activity and targeted multifactorial interventions. Further progress will be made if large-scale randomized controlled trials are conducted that can confirm the effectiveness of these interventions and examine other interventions suggested from observational studies.

REFERENCES

1 Sloane PD, Dallara J. Clinical research and geriatric dizziness: the blind men and the elephant. *Journal of the American Geriatrics Society* 1999; 47: 113–14.

2 Liu YJ, Stagni G, Walden JG, Shepherd AMM, Lichtenstein MJ. Thioridazine dose-related effects on biomechanical force platform measures of sway in young and old men. *Journal of the American Geriatrics Society* 1998; 46: 431–7.

3 Nevitt M, Cummings S, Kidd S, Black D. Risk factors for recurrent nonsyncopal falls. *Journal of the American Medical Association* 1989; 261: 2663–8.

4 Shumway-Cook A, Woollacott M, Kerns KA, Baldwin, M. The effects of two types of cognitive tasks on postural stability in older adults with and without a history of falls. *Journals of Gerontology: Biological and Medical Sciences* 1997; 52: M232–40.

5 Lord SR, Matters BR, Corcoran JM, Howland AS, Fitzpatrick RC. Choice reaction time stepping: a composite measure of the risk of falling in older people. *Gait and Posture* 1999; 9: S29.

6 Lord SR, Ward JA, Williams P, Anstey K. Physiological factors associated with falls in older community-dwelling women. *Journal of the American Geriatrics Society* 1994;42:1110–17.

7 Lundin-Olsson L, Nyberg L, Gustafson Y. 'Stops walking while talking' as a predictor of falls in elderly people. *Lancet* 1997; 349: 617.

8 Province MA, Hadley EC, Hornbrook MC, et al. The effects of exercise on falls in elderly patients. A preplanned meta-analysis of the FICSIT Trials. Frailty and injuries: cooperative studies of intervention techniques. *Journal of the American Medical Association* 1995; 273: 1341–7.

9 Cumming R, Thomas M, Szonyi G, et al. Home visits by an occupational therapist for assessment and modification of environmental hazards: a randomized controlled trial of falls prevention. *Journal of the American Geriatrics Society* 1999; 47:1397–1402.

10 Campbell AJ, Robertson MC, Gardner MM, Norton RN, Buchner DM. Psychotropic medication withdrawal and a home-based exercise programme to prevent falls: a randomized controlled trial. *Journal of the American Geriatrics Society* 1999; 47: 850–3.

11 Wolf-Klein GP, Silverstone FA, Basavaraju N, Foley CJ, Pascaru A, Ma PH. Prevention of falls in the elderly population. *Archives of Physical Medicine and Rehabilitation* 1988; 6: 689–91.

12 Hill KD, Dwyer JM, Schwarz JA, Helme RD. A falls and balance clinic for the elderly. *Physiotherapy Canada* 1994; 46: 20–27.

Index